Success in
Veterinary
Practice

Success in Veterinary Practice

Maximizing Clinical Outcomes and Personal Well-Being

Dr Bradley Viner
BVetMed MSc(VetGP) DProf MRCVS

WILEY-BLACKWELL

A John Wiley & Sons, Ltd., Publication

Wiley-Blackwell is an imprint of John Wiley & Sons, formed by the merger of Wiley's global Scientific, Technical and Medical business with Blackwell Publishing.

Registered office
John Wiley & Sons Ltd, The Atrium, Southern Gate, Chichester, West Sussex, PO19 8SQ, United Kingdom

Editorial offices
9600 Garsington Road, Oxford, OX4 2DQ, United Kingdom
2121 State Avenue, Ames, Iowa 50014-8300, USA

For details of our global editorial offices, for customer services and for information about how to apply for permission to reuse the copyright material in this book please see our website at www.wiley.com/wiley-blackwell.

Library of Congress Cataloging-in-Publication Data

Viner, Bradley.
  Success in veterinary practice : maximising clinical outcomes and personal well-being / Bradley Viner.
     p. ; cm.
  Includes bibliographical references and index.
  ISBN 978-1-4051-6950-9 (pbk. : alk. paper)
  1. Veterinary medicine–Practice. I. Title.
  [DNLM: 1. Practice Management–organization & administration.
2. Veterinary Medicine–organization & administration.   3. Hospitals, Animal.
SF 756.4 V782s 2009]
  SF756.4.V56 2009
  636.089'0695–dc22   2009024486

A catalogue record for this book is available from the British Library.

Set in 10/13pt Palatino by Aptara® Inc., New Delhi, India
Printed and bound in Malaysia by KHL Printing Co Sdn Bhd

1   2010

Contents

Acknowledgements

Although this book took a couple of years to research and write, it was founded upon 30 years of work in veterinary general practice. I have been fortunate through that time to have worked with some first-class colleagues, and I thank them all for the support and inspiration that they have given to me over the years. Teamwork is essential to good veterinary practice, and I have indeed been fortunate in the team that I have been able to gather around me.

My work with what began as my MSc learning set and developed into a doctoral group has spanned five enjoyable and challenging years of my life. Learning and researching out of interest rather than necessity has been a helter-skelter of extreme highs and deep lows, and the peer support of other members of my group has become a highly valued part of my life. I consider myself fortunate to have been involved with such a talented and warm-hearted group of vets, but even more surprised by all the efforts that others from outside the profession have been prepared to offer in terms of support and encouragement. Professor David Lane and Dr Annette Fillery-Travis of the Professional Development Foundation have given countless hours of their time to support our group, well over and above the call of duty and I thank them wholeheartedly.

As my doctoral work developed, I spent increasing amounts of time working with the members of the clinical audit MSc group, and was able to facilitate the formation of a new learning set. Although the experience was as new to them as it had been to my own MSc group before, they soon found their feet and blossomed impressively. They contributed far more to the development of guidelines for the introduction of clinical audit into the profession than I could have on my own. I am very grateful for all their input, their friendship and for their permission base much of Chapter 4 upon work that was produced collaboratively.

Whenever I have sought advice from outside sources, or requested permission to quote a piece of work, I have always been given assistance and encouragement. There are too many people to mention individually, but I am indebted to them all. Any comments that have been made have been reflected upon, and where appropriate, my text has been modified.

I must give a special thanks to all my family, who have been so supportive when my literary efforts have made me into a distracted and antisocial member of the family. I am painfully aware that even when I have not been writing, it has sometimes been all too obvious that my thoughts have been elsewhere. I am immensely proud of both my children: Oliver, who has taken the step that I hope he will never regret and followed me into veterinary general practice; and Emma, who has just submitted her thesis for a professional doctorate whilst working in the immensely stimulating and worthwhile profession of educational psychology. And finally to my darling wife, Liz, who has remained loyally supportive through all my efforts. After more than 30 years of marriage I still love her more than ever.

Bradley Viner
May 2009

Introduction

The first principle is that you must not fool yourself - and you are the easiest person to fool. Richard Feynman (Nobel Laureate physicist)

IS THIS THE BOOK FOR YOU?

Perhaps you are reading this introduction before you have made up your mind to purchase, borrow, or pinch this book, so let me give you some advice that may help you with your decision on whether this is the one for you:

- If you are looking for a practice management book that will simply tell you how to run a veterinary practice, this one won't fit the bill: there are excellent veterinary management books on the market.
- If you are looking for a book that will tell you all the answers as to how you, as a veterinarian, should be running your professional life, you won't find your answers in any book. You have to look to yourself for those answers, but this book is designed to guide you to go through the process.
- If you are a grumpy old man (or woman) who treats any book aimed at self-improvement with contempt, then you should definitely purchase a copy: you won't learn anything from it,

but you will be able to gain countless hours of enjoyment from deriding its content.

This is not a book about managing a good veterinary practice, but a book about managing ourselves as veterinarians. It is primarily aimed at the veterinary profession, but may also be of interest to those that work closely with that most peculiar of species and would benefit from understanding more about what makes us tick. Or not. Parts would be very valuable to those undergoing veterinary undergraduate training, or just contemplating embarking on such a career.

Most veterinarians are good at responding to what is thrown at us, because we are trained to try and meet the urgent needs of our clients and their charges. We are generally much poorer at dealing with all the less urgent issues that can be put aside in the short term, but are every bit as important to our long term careers. This book aims to help us find a space in our lives to consider the issues that need to be dealt with on a proactive basis, to provide ourselves with a clear vision of what we want to get out of our professional careers, and how best to get there.

WHY IS THIS BOOK NECESSARY?

Those of us working within the veterinary profession are the envy of many others in society. How often do we hear the statement "You're so lucky. I always wanted to work with animals – I still do, but (for one reason or another) I was not able to make it to veterinary school"?

We have fought to gain acceptance onto one of the most sought after and competitive degree courses; we have overcome the not inconsiderable hurdles that the undergraduate course throws at us; and we have entered a profession with a wide choice of stimulating and worthwhile career paths. So why waste time contemplating our navels?

Whilst there are undoubtedly members of the profession that sail through their careers leading fulfilled and satisfied lives, the statistics suggest that the garden is not all quite as rosy. A considerable number of studies, summarized by Bartram and

Baldwin (2007a), have shown that veterinarians in a wide range of countries, including the US, UK, Australia and Norway, have the highest rate of suicide of any profession. It is generally agreed to be twice that of other health professionals, and four times that of dentists. Burnout is also common, with many practitioners becoming disillusioned with the stresses and rewards that general practice can offer, and leaving the profession to follow different careers paths (Elkins and Elkins, 1987). It seems that the great aspirations held by those planning to enter the profession are all too often not matched by the reality of their lives after graduation, leading to disillusionment and depression. One of the major themes of this book is that time spent on reflection is very rarely time wasted – we always manage to find the time to put things right that have gone wrong because we have rushed into them, often causing us considerable stress in the process. We can save a lot more time in the long run by pausing before rushing into the early stages of a project to contemplate issues such as:

- Why am I carrying it out?
- How important is it to me?
- Does it conflict with any of my core values?
- Should I be taking it on at all, and if so, how best can I approach it?

This enables us to be proactive rather just responsive to the demands that are placed upon us.

If we learn to become more mindful of what we are doing, we can direct our energies in the most effective manner. We can also develop a greater understanding of what motivates us, and how and why we react emotionally to the issues that face us. In turn, that can help us to generate the maximum happiness from the work that we do – not just short-term pleasure, but the deeper and more lasting satisfaction that working as part of a highly effective veterinary team can bring.

WHO IS QUALIFIED TO HELP GUIDE PRACTITIONERS?

Primary care has traditionally been taught by specialists employed in the veterinary faculties, who typically have a great deal of knowledge about their subject area but precious little experience of applying them in a general practice setting. This is changing within the medical profession, with teaching commonly being taken out into practice, but within the veterinary context this is much less formalized. Medical primary care training also now deals with many more issues than clinical care alone. Although there are many books and articles that have been written about important personal subjects such as motivation, values and learning, few of them have been set within a veterinary scenario. Bartram and Boniwell (2007b) recently reviewed happiness and psychological well-being within the veterinary profession and concluded that they are determined more by our state of mind than our external conditions, and can be achieved through reshaping attitudes and outlook. It would seem that guidance in areas such as these could bring key benefits to our working lives, yet it is outside the scope of our usual postgraduate learning.

As mature professionals we need to develop the confidence to identify our *own* learning needs and then seek out the best means of meeting them. The intensity of the veterinary undergraduate course invariably encourages a 'spoon-feeding' mentality where we are most comfortable when we are sitting back and being fed with the information that we need to know – ready to regurgitate it on command. The answers to the major questions that this book will raise are personal to you, and the answers are within you if you only make the decision to seek them out. That doesn't mean that they are always simple, or even easy to find. We think we know ourselves, yet once we begin to delve we discover that we are often our own worst enemies: we lie to ourselves, we hide issues from ourselves and we make surprisingly bad snap judgements about ourselves. Being honest with ourselves and bringing such issues out into the open can be difficult and deeply troubling, but well worth the effort in the long run.

MY JOURNEY

I'm going to begin by telling you a little about the path of own veterinary career, towards a goal of identifying and helping to develop the specific skills that practicing veterinarians need to develop in order to thrive. I can claim some plausibility as a role model, having established a thriving group of five veterinary practices on the outskirts of London, but as always, there is as much to be learnt from the errors I have made along the way as from the successes. Maybe one measure of my success has been that my son Oliver was sufficiently impressed by the style of life that veterinary practice has brought to me to have decided to join the profession himself. He is currently a recent graduate, and it is too early to say if he will regret his decision, but the signs are encouraging. If at any stage in this book my tone becomes patronising, I beg forgiveness on the basis that it is inevitable that some of the time I should lapse into giving the advice that a father would wish to pass on to his son as he sets out to make his own mark in the profession.

Professional learning is a journey, although often we have little idea of where it will take us. My personal journey of formalized postgraduate education began back in 2001, when I had already been working in small animal veterinary practice for over 20 years, and I was well on my way to establishing the network of clinics that presently own. Up until then my veterinary professional development had followed a fairly traditional path, attending veterinary conventions and meetings once or twice a year, and a potpourri of lectures and seminars on subjects that tickled my interest. I had noticed an increasing propensity to fall gently asleep once the lights were dimmed, and very few of the sessions that I attended actually ended up changing the way that I did things when I returned to my practice.

Then, in response to an advertisement, I joined a group of eight veterinarians who all felt strongly that it was time to establish the first qualification in veterinary general practice in the UK. We found ourselves under the wing of Professor David Lane and the National Centre for Work-based Learning at the University of Middlesex. There is a Zen Buddhist saying that

When the pupil is ready, the master appears.

It does indeed seem fortunate that we were paired with such an excellent mentor at a time in our careers when we were receptive to change. We had some idea about where we wanted to end up, but no concept of the route that we would take to get there. Professor Lane had very little experience of the world of veterinary practice, but his work developing frameworks of competence to drive and appraise the postgraduate training of clinical psychologists, made him the ideal person to guide us along our way.

Seven years on, all eight of the original group completed MSc degrees with the University of Middlesex, studying different aspects of postgraduate education for practicing veterinarians, and four have gone on to complete Professional Doctorates, researching selected areas in more depth. The Royal College of Veterinary Surgeons, the body that oversees postgraduate veterinary education in the UK, launched their new postgraduate modular Certificates, and many of the concepts put forwards by our group have been incorporated into the final model. This includes an option to study for the RCVS Advanced Certificate in Veterinary General Practice, alongside options for the more traditional specialties such as Dermatology, Orthopaedics and Production Animal Medicine.

It sounds so simple when I summarize the work of our group in a couple of paragraphs, that it seems ridiculous that when we started out, the hurdles seemed almost insurmountable. Despite the fact that primary care is now well recognized as a specialty within medical practice, the concept of a postgraduate qualification in veterinary general practice was coming up against a brick wall from experienced general practitioners:

How can you become more specialized *in general practice?*
The skills that you need are what students are taught at veterinary school anyway!
Exactly who *is qualified to tell* us *what we should be doing in our own practices?*

It has always seemed obvious to me there *are* specific skills that need to be finely honed to excel in general veterinary practice. In recent years the veterinary schools have become more mindful of the need to teach the 'softer' para-clinical skills as well as the more obvious clinical ones. Just as the basic dermatology, that is taught at an undergraduate level can be strengthened by postgraduate learning, so can competences such as communication skills, team working and the measurement and maintenance of standards of clinical effectiveness. The development of such competences is just as important to the outcome of a particular case as the underlying clinical knowledge. You may be brimming over with clinical information about a particular case, but if you and your team are unable to get an owner onside with you to carry out an agreed course of treatment, you will have to rely upon your patient getting better *in spite* of your assistance rather than *because* of it. Just because such skills may be harder to teach and to assess, does not mean that they are any less important in terms of a successful veterinary career. Indeed, if we look at the areas that commonly cause professional problems, or perhaps even a change to another career path, a lack of clinical knowledge does not usually figure among them.

I was raised within the educational paradigm where teachers told students what they needed to know, and the measure of academic success was the ability to reproduce that information in an exam situation. The accumulation of knowledge is a necessary part of professional learning, but there is a strong argument to suggest that the old paradigm actually resulted in a narrowing of students' horizons and thought processes, making them less fit for the task that would face them after graduation rather than more so. This is even truer for postgraduate learning, where it is the successful application of knowledge within the workplace that should be the measure of its success.

Members of my postgraduate learning group did have a destination in our minds to help drive us forwards, and we were very fortunate to have some very effective mentors to guide us along the way. But we all found that we gained just as much from the journey itself, as compared to any success that we achieved in reaching our objectives. We discovered a great deal about the tools that could be used to help support professional learning, such as the vital importance of reflective practice, and the power of action learning, where members of a learning set help each other to probe the issues that are barriers to their progress. Most importantly, we discovered how mature professionals can work to develop their own learning objectives, that are most closely related to their personal goals, and then develop their own route towards fulfilling them. There is nothing new in these concepts within the wider professional spectrum, but veterinary practitioners have traditionally been very hung up on relying on others to tell them what they think they need to know.

The aim of this book is to help you define your own measure of successful practice, identify the traits and skills required, and work out how to encourage the development and practical application of those skills. Quality of care will obviously come into the equation, but it has to be balanced with a quality of life that is likely to provide you with the physical and mental health that you require to maintain those long-term standards.

Rather than providing answers, much of it raises questions; questions that will hopefully help you to think more closely about what you do how you do it, why you do it, and most importantly, how you could do it better. It is aimed to help provide the tools to enable you to fathom out the answers to these crucial questions, because it is only by reflecting upon these issues within your own workplace that you can come up with solutions that are truly relevant to your needs.

What I and other members of our learning group discovered was both very simple and yet completely revolutionary, turning each of our own world views on its head. In this book, I aim to take what is most useful from a whole range of professional learning and management disciplines and apply them to the veterinary scenario. I am confident that my conclusions are relevant to veterinarians in any type of practice in just about any part of the world, because the concepts involved are truly universal ones. I am not a trained psychologist or educationalist, but there is a great deal that I have learned by looking outside the veterinary 'box' from the viewpoint of someone firmly grounded in veterinary practice that is worth attempting to pass on to other members of this fine profession.

Bradley Viner
May 2009

Caring about Quality

Quality is not an act. It is a habit. (Aristotle, 384 BC–322 BC).

This book is founded upon the assumption that success in veterinary practice depends upon two things:

Premise One

Long term financial success will follow on from efficiently providing a high quality of client and patient care appropriate to the particular sector or sectors in which the practice is operating.

Premise Two

Whilst financial success can provide a short term basis for our motivation and well-being, long term satisfaction is only likely to be achieved if there is harmony between our personal values and goals and our professional objectives, and we are content with the place that our profession occupies within our lives.

You might take issue with those assumptions, perhaps believing it is possible to get what you want out of life by providing a poor quality service at a very competitive price, working very long hours and possibly making lots of money. That is your prerogative, as there will always be a market for a low cost, high turnover style of practice, but it is my firm belief that good medicine is good business, and is the path most likely to lead to a satisfactory work/life balance and long-term personal well-being.

This chapter picks up this theme by attempting to establish what quality care actually means, before moving on in later chapters to consider how that can be enhanced and set within the overall context of a rewarding life as a veterinarian.

Surprisingly, up until now no one has tried to do this in any formalized way within the context of the veterinary profession, but it is something that has occupied a considerable amount of academic reflection in other fields.

BEST PRACTICE AND CLINICAL EXCELLENCE

Is quality care simply about applying 'best practice' to every clinical case? Best practice is a recognized management concept used widely in industry and commerce as well as the health professions which asserts that there is a technique which is more effective at delivering a particular outcome than any other. Best practice can also be defined as the most **efficient** (involving the least amount of effort or expense) and **effective** (producing the best results) way of accomplishing a task.

It is interesting to consider the extent to which best practice can be generalized from one workplace to another. For example, a group of specialists might formulate 'Best Practice Guidelines for the Investigation and Treatment of Syncope in Dogs' that they feel outline the ideal approach to investigating and treating this particular clinical condition. Their conclusions may be soundly evidence-based and stand up well to critical analysis, but a primary care practitioner who attempts to slavishly impose the full gamut of tests upon every case that is brought in through the consulting room door is likely to run into problems. Ideally, the clinician's actions should be informed by knowledge of what best practice actually is for this type of case, but good veterinary care is something that needs to be guided by common sense, tempering the goal of a clinical ideal with an intimate knowledge of the local situation and the individual patient and its owner. Arguably, your best practice is what works best in your particular workplace.

Applying best practice clinically is only one part of the larger picture that describes the range of issues that need to be addressed to provide an optimal service to our patients and their owners. It also implies that excellence is a fixed objective that can be achieved, whereas I am firmly of the view that it is a moving goalpost, and that however well we do something, we can always find a way of doing it just that little bit better. More of that in Chapter 4.

Exercise – Perceptions of Excellence in Practice

Excellence means different things to different people, and seeing those issues from differing viewpoints helps us to reflect upon what is important for us to develop.

Draw up a simple grid. Along the top put five people:

- Yourself
- A client
- A key member of your practice's staff
- A junior member of your practice's staff
- Your partner or an important member of your family

Number the horizontal columns one to five, and list what you consider each would consider to be the most important characteristics that would enable them to recognize good veterinary practice. Then highlight the differences between your own viewpoint and theirs so that you can reflect upon them and decide if they make you feel you would wish to change your own priorities in any way. You might even like to carry out a mini-survey of the people concerned to see if their opinions match the views that you ascribe to them. You may be surprised at the results.

A LOOK IN THE MIRROR

A term which has become unfashionable these days is *calling*, yet the concept still underlies what having a meaningful vocation signifies. Indeed, the term *vocation* is based upon the Latin word meaning 'to be called', suggesting that a good worker has been singled out and called to carry out their work by a higher authority. Howard Gardner, Mihaly Csikszentmihalyi (which out of interest is pronounced chick-sent-me-high) and William Damon are highly respected professors of psychology who have written a book that summarizes their major joint project entitled *Good Work* (Gardner et al., 2006), which examines the essence of excellence in a selected profession. They have suggested that this ancient concept of a calling can be framed in a more contemporary fashion by the psychological concept of moral identity, which is what a professional experiences when they think about themselves and their occupation in moral terms. If a professional has strived to do what they consider to be the right thing, and live up to the values that drove them to take up their vocation in the first place, they will be able to look at themselves in the mirror and like what they see, metaphorically, at least. If the sense of calling degenerates into just another job, a way of keeping food on the plate and the BMW in the garage, the moral identity slips away and the mirror sends back a less attractive image.

A Short Exercise in Self-Image

Look at yourself face to face in a mirror. Do it, don't just imagine it. Question yourself about what you do, how you do it, what motivates you, how you feel about your life, about yourself. Try and look at yourself not as 'you' but as someone observing yourself, so that you can 'see' the emotions that you are feeling dispassion-ately. Try not to get caught up in them – so for example, if you are angry or remorseful about something, look at that emotion and observe what it feels like to experience it.

Contrary to the advice in the previous section, try not to make value judgements about what you observe, just try to see yourself as you are. We think we know ourselves, we think we are honest with ourselves, but the reality is that we become so wrapped up with living life and with the flow of motions that run through our bodies, that we often end up with a very poor self-awareness. Positive change in our behaviour will often follow naturally once we start taking time to get to know ourselves and understand the thoughts and emotions that drive us.

THE FOUNDATIONS OF GOOD VETERINARY PRACTICE

Howard Gardner and his colleagues at the Good Work Project have attempted to crystallize the four key elements that they con-sider to lay the foundations of good work in our time. Whether a person does good, compromised or poor work they see as the result of at least four major forces, which can be adapted for ap-plication to the veterinary profession (Figure 1.1):

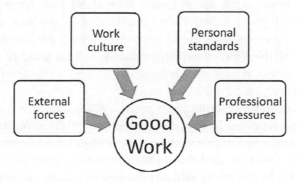

Figure 1.1 Pressures on good work in veterinary practice.

Personal standards include our values, beliefs and self-image. They are based upon genetic traits, early experiences, values learned in the family, but may be modified by both social and cultural controls. Our views of society's relationships with animals are particularly relevant.

Work culture is the demands of our own veterinary practice, and how clearly they are stated: what constitutes good performance, and how that can best be obtained.

External forces influence attitudes to our work. For example, if there is a shortage of supply of veterinarians, our work may be more highly valued, or in times of oversupply we may feel more obliged to bow to commercial pressures. External events such as disease outbreaks may also affect how the public see our role.

Professional pressures emanate from others working within the veterinary profession at large. Hopefully they are well aligned with external attitudes to our work, but sometimes there is a conflict between the two, and what is expected in practice differs from what broader society expects.

Howard Gardner and his colleagues conclude that 'Good Work' is likely to occur when there are clear and strong standards for what constitutes desirable performance: standards that are enforced by a concerned professional community; standards that are internalized in the self-image of practitioners; and standards that are not contradicted by strong external pressure from market, political, or social forces. If all these four types of controls are aligned, 'Good Work' is probable. If the four controls pull in different directions, or one or more are absent, it is likely that the kind of work produced will be shoddy at best, and at worst it will be detrimental to the well-being of the community.

This could be described as a practice ethos, which is framed so that those working in that environment are clear about their objectives and comfortable with how those objectives sit within their own value system, and that of their broader community. Fostering such a harmonious ethos is the key to success in veterinary practice.

HALLMARKS OF EXCELLENCE

Another way of looking at the development of good veterinary practice would be to attempt to identify the character traits that are thought to be most closely related to a high level of performance as a practitioner. In his book, *The Inner Apprentice*, experienced medical practitioner and tutor Roger Neighbour (2005) carried out a survey of GP medical training course organizers, asking them to identify what they considered to be hallmarks of medical excellence in the postgraduate students that passed through their hands. Their responses were organized into groups and ranked as follows:

- Positive response to novelty (41%)
- A caring attitude (40%)
- Up-to-date clinical competence (37%)
- Self-awareness (35%)
- Group ability (34%)
- Personal qualities (30%)
- Educability (29%)
- Motivation (28%)
- Balance (20%)
- Industry (19%)
- Communication skills (16%)
- Mission (15%)
- Critical ability (7%)
- Diversity (7%)

This crude estimation is a long way from definitively identifying the personality traits that are most important to producing a highly competent veterinarian. Firstly, they only apply to medical graduates, although it is not unreasonable to assume that there will be a strong correlation between the two professions. More importantly, they are based upon opinions expressed by one group of people, albeit those with considerable experience of postgraduate medical training and its outcomes. A most robust approach would be to measure the character traits of new medical graduates using one of the many psychometric tools that are available, and then after a suitable interval, comparing those results to their success in practice. Yet even this approach would pose problems, for how does one objectively measure the all-round competence of a practitioner? Would it be by a 360-degree survey of their work colleagues, a survey of their patients, or even the stage that their career had advanced after a set amount of time? All would be open to criticism, so perhaps the opinions of a group of experienced practitioner-tutors are not such a poor option after all.

Some of the results that Neighbour uncovered are surprising. Who would have thought that a positive attitude to novelty would top the list, above a caring attitude and clinical knowledge? The benefits of positivity as a psychological stance are a key message in the later chapters of this book. This must be closely linked to the traits of motivation and educability that come further down the list, but Neighbour maintains that educators see the ability to relish the unknown rather than fear it as being crucial to success in practice.

Personal and team skills such as self-awareness and the ability to work within a group rate highly in the list, but the ranking of communication skills outside the top ten is somewhat contrary to expectation.

There is little doubt that the selection and training of veterinary undergraduates is geared towards the development of clinical competence, and that is not an area that should be ignored. But we have to ask how well does conventional training encourage the other qualities in the list? There is a common misapprehension that these are traits that you either possess or not – that they can't be learnt. But a great deal of research (Silverman et al., 2004) has shown that although individuals may vary in their intrinsic abilities within these areas, training can bring about a significant improvement in performance.

Exercise in Self-Development

Take the list of character traits above and consider whether how far you agree with their relative importance. Are there others you feel are not covered by the list? Consider how do you rate yourself against each of those traits, and what steps, if any, you feel you could take to develop them further, particularly those where you feel you rate relatively poorly.

THE QUALITY OF VETERINARY PRACTICE

We have looked at the input side of good veterinary practice – the characteristics that an individual needs to foster in order to become highly competent, but we also need to look at the output – just what do we mean by a high quality of care, and how can we measure it?

We tend to think that we know what we mean by the term 'quality', but it is not an absolute, and there are different ways of interpreting it. Garvin (1984) defines five categories:

1. Transcendent: The most common usage out of the sphere of business, with quality seen as the absolute degree of excellence and associated with premium products such as Rolls Royce or the Ritz Hotel. It does not take account of the fact that less prestigious suppliers can still provide a quality product, albeit at a different level.
2. Product-based: Quality is a descriptor of the product being sold, such as for carpets, which might be 'bedroom quality' or 'living room quality' – suitable for a particular purpose.
3. Manufacturing-based: Conformance to a specification set by the supplier. This may not be the same as what the customer expects. This is similar to a veterinarian who defines quality without reference to a client's experiences and wishes.
4. User (consumer)-based: Involves meeting the expectations of the customer, but does not explicitly take account of the costs involved.
5. Value-based: Quality is defined not as what is 'best' in absolute terms, but that which establishes the optimum balance between cost and the value of the service to the client. This definition is of more relevance to businesses operating in the non-premium sector of the market, and carries a danger of using its competitive pricing to justify providing the consumer with a lower quality than is actually desired.

Within the medical sphere, Moullin (2002) proposes the most appropriate definition to be 'meeting customer requirements and expectations at an acceptable price', which is actually a hybrid of the consumer-based and value-based definitions. In his forward to 'Professional Development in General Practice' (Pendleton and Hasler, 1997), Professor David Metcalf, professor of general practice at the University of Manchester defines four components of high quality medical care that can be easily extended to the veterinary context:

1. It must be safe.
2. It must be humane – considerate of the feelings of the patient, or in our case, both the patient and its owner.
3. It must be as effective as possible.
4. It must be economic – this is even more true of veterinary practice, where we have a client directly paying for the cost of care.

Another dimension that is increasingly being recognized is the need for services to be client-centred. For example, Harr (2001) carried out a survey in Switzerland to investigate why patients changed their dentist, and discovered that only 15% did so on the basis of cost or poor quality of work, and 70% gave the reason as poor service or lack of courtesy among the practice staff. It would seem that this is very relevant to the competitive veterinary market. A survey carried out in the US in 1999 identified caring and kindness, respectful treatment and 'informativeness' as the most important factors guiding their choice of a veterinarian (Brown and Silverman, 1999).

Some Tips for Client-Centredness in Veterinary Practice

- Give clients control over the treatment that their pet receives. This involves providing information about its illness, and alternative options for treatment.
- Integrate services across professions. We need to retain professional supervision of the veterinary care that their patient receives, but should be prepared to work with other

professionals such as behaviourists and physiotherapists to obtain the optimum results.

- Consider the 'client's experience' in terms of the practice environment, waiting times and accessibility.
- Prioritize the continuity of veterinary care.
- Consider the courtesy and efficiency of the staff that come into contact with the client.
- Aim to provide a fair and equitable service, including making all reasonable efforts to assist clients with disabilities.

The list of what customers of Nissan UK said that they wanted (David, 1990) can be equally well applied to veterinary practice:

- Don't ignore me.
- Make me feel wanted.
- Don't lie to me.
- Give me clear information.
- Don't insult my intelligence.
- Keep your promises.
- Don't keep me waiting.
- Listen to me when I tell you how to improve your services.
- Be sensitive to my needs.
- Treat me fairly – don't rip me off.
- And the one he forgot – be nice to my dog.

Achieving Quality: Ten Objectives for Veterinary Practice

Traditionally, quality control has simply looked at the output of a process, and identified any that come below par – in the case of manufacturing say, an item of clothing, it is simple enough to discard any products that do not come up to the required quality, or sell them off more cheaply as seconds. This concept is not nearly as appealing when we are dealing with patients, be they human or animal.

The concept of total quality management (TQM) was originally developed to supervise manufacturing output, but was adapted for medical health care by Donald Berwick (1989) at the Institute of Health Care Improvement in Boston. It aims to look at every stage of a process and to try and optimize performance, rather than just maintain it above a minimum standard. Berwick identified the following objectives for organizational change that are required to enable TQM, and they can readily be applied to veterinary practice:

1. Focusing on quality – the practice needs to have a strategy dedicated to quality improvement and be capable of organizing it within a realistic time frame.
2. A committed leadership, not just at practice partner level, but within each aspect of the clinical team. This will be developed further in Chapter 6.
3. Client-minded, monitoring and responding to the needs of clients when introducing changes within the practice.
4. Employee-minded, improving working conditions and listening to staff's information and views, thus enabling them to fulfil their potential.
5. Process-minded, looking at the systems that have been set up as a framework for the workforce, rather than trying to apportion individual blame.
6. Statistically minded, measuring performance before and after changes has been put into place, in order to identify problems and confirm their improvement. This will be developed further in Chapter 3.
7. Dedicated to continuous improvement, so that the processes that we put into place operate continually rather than spasmodically (see below).
8. Treating suppliers as partners, such as affording drug company representatives with respect in order to allow them to offer the best service that they can.
9. Innovative, using vision to make changes and achieve improvement, rather than just patching up what already exists.
10. Proactive, showing a determination to be the best rather than just maintaining a satisfactory level of performance.

So, here we have the essence of how good veterinary practice can be put into effect at an organizational level, but putting such a strategy into place requires a serious commitment to providing the highest quality of care throughout the veterinary team. We shall return to the subject of clinical governance and the quality of veterinary clinical care in Chapter 4.

Continuous Improvement in Veterinary Health Care

Donald Berwick (1989) describes two approaches to quality improvement in health care, the first of which he calls the Theory of Bad Apples, or quality by inspection, which measures output with a view to rooting out workers that fail to perform to a required standard. The long-term effect is usually to drag down performance to what is considered to be an acceptable level, rather than push it upwards.

The Theory of Continuous Improvement was developed in Japanese industry as a positive tool to drive standards upwards, and it is equally applicable to a veterinary practice of any size. It is based on *kaizen* – the continuous search for opportunities to get better, and starts with the contrary premise to the Theory of Bad Apples that workers do fundamentally care about the quality of the work that they carry out. This is probably more true in human and animal health care than in any other area of work. Problems that lead to poor performance usually relate to the systems that have been put into place, and even when human resources are the cause, it is usually because of poor job design, poor leadership, or unclear purpose. This paradigm is captured in the phrase 'Every defect is treasured', because it is only by uncovering defects that processes can be improved. This approach has been shown to deliver results. For example, Xerox engineers visiting Japan in 1979 found copiers being produced at half the cost of those manufactured by them in the US, with only 1/30th the number of defects.

The Cost of Quality

It might be assumed that quality costs more, yet the relationship is not so clear-cut – bad quality also costs money. Most improvements in quality do require extra investment of one sort or another, but many also produce long-term cost benefits. When considering the cost of instituting changes that affect quality, the following elements need to be considered:

Costs of quality control:

1. Cost of prevention: If we take the example of reducing post-operative infection rates, perhaps sterile gowns, gloves and masks might be introduced at an extra cost. Even if no extra consumables are used, the process of holding meetings to identify areas to improve, writing guidelines and additional training all carry a cost.
2. Cost of appraisal: Auditing the quality of the output, in this case postoperative infection rates, and then monitoring performance to determine any change is an essential part of a quality management framework, but carries a cost in terms of the staff time and training involved.

Costs of *not* having effective quality control:

1. Internal failure costs: The resources involved in rectifying a service that was performed incorrectly but does not directly affect the service user. For instance, if case data was not recorded properly, then significant amounts of time may be wasted trying to track down who carried out the procedure and exactly what was done, in order to try and pinpoint a cause.
2. External failure costs: The costs of mistakes that directly affect our clients. Sometimes these cannot be put right after the event, and cause a devastating effect upon the animals involved and upon staff morale. At other times they may be more easily quantifiable, such as the cost of additional medical treatment or even surgery that has to be carried out to correct the problem. Dealing with complaints, and possible litigation, add an extra element of cost in some instances.

The cost of preventing problems may be relatively low, but the cost of avoiding the necessary action to attend to issues of quality may be high and unavoidable. Problems arise when there is a significant gap between the level of service that a client expects, and that which they receive. There are several possible reasons why such a gap may exist:

1. A lack of awareness of precisely what clients expect.
2. An awareness of what clients want, but a conscious decision not to take the appropriate action to provide that particular standard of service.
3. A knowledge of what level of service to provide, but an inability to deliver it because of staff issues such as inadequate training or poor communications.
4. Client's expectations that may have been raised to an unrealistic level by the claims made about the service offered.

These barriers to meeting client's expectations can exist either at an individual level, in the consulting room, or at an organizational level across a practice. It is essential to recognize if an expectation gap is occurring, and why, before steps can be taken to remedy it.

Exercise – The First Steps

A journey of a thousand miles begins with a single step. (Zen Buddhist proverb)

1. Look at the list of ten objectives for organizational change outlined by Berwick above. Use them as a basis for identifying ten things you could do now to improve the quality of care that you could offer. Feel free to stray outside the box if other sources of inspiration spring to mind. Each individual action should be relatively minor and easily achievable.
2. Consider carefully how many do you think you could realistically manage to put into effect – not some nebulous time in the future, but now. Three? Perhaps five. Don't be overambitious, because you can always come back for more.
3. Look down the list that you have made and prioritize them in order of those that you think will be most beneficial to your practice.
4. Plan how you will put each into effect, using the SMART mnemonic to help you:

Significant
Measurable
Achievable
Relevant
Timed

Consider how you can get your practice team involved with each area, so that they buy in to what is being done. Better still, involve them in the decision-making process.

5.   Now get stuck in and put them into effect, but set up a reminder on your online organizer or mobile phone to remind you to review your progress at the end of the time you have specified.

Providing a quality service does not come from any single intervention, but from a large number of small changes that have to become inculcated into the culture of your practice. Neither should you ever reach a quality of care that fully satisfies you, for with satisfaction will come complacency. Continual improvement needs to become a way of life, so this process should become part of your management routine.

ACHIEVING BALANCE: THREE PROFESSIONAL COMPETENCIES

Success in veterinary practice isn't just about doing one thing really well, or even about doing everything possible to perfection, because that veterinary nirvana simply does not exist. It is more about gaining an understanding of the various areas of our personal and professional development and by developing our self-awareness, balancing them so that they work together harmoniously.

The areas of professional competence can broadly be divided into three:

1.   Clinical ability, which is largely knowledge-based, but also involves some specific physical skills, such as surgical competence, or the ability to use certain diagnostic tools ranging

from ophthalmoscopes through to ultrasound machines, and to interpret the information they provide. Veterinary undergraduate and postgraduate training has a tendency to focus upon this area, partly because it underpins our professional activities, but also because its teaching and assessment is relatively straightforward and familiar. A postgraduate approach to optimizing clinical effectiveness is outlined in Chapter 4.

2. Interpersonal skills, which determine our ability to interface effectively with our clients, their animals, those that share our workplace, and with the professional world at large. Animal handling has always been an integral part of every veterinary curriculum, but interpersonal skills have only recently become incorporated into the courses, and many of us in practice will have received little or no formal training in those areas. Communications is dealt with in Chapter 5.

3. Personal skills, which determine how we manage our own lives. Some of these have an obvious relevance to our ability to perform in our work, such as an awareness of how we learn, and how our personality type interfaces with others. Others, such as how we occupy our time away from work and cope with the stresses that confront us, have traditionally been seen as private, and as 'true professionals', not allowed to impinge upon our work. In reality, we are all affected by our lives away from our practices, and often wrestle to try and reconcile the two. Finding the optimum balance between our work and the rest of our lives will have some effect upon our short-term performance, but will have a major effect upon our ability to thrive in practice in the long term (Fig 1.2).

Have a think now about how you rate yourself in each of these areas. Much of the rest of the book will be taken up with the development of personal skills, as this is the most neglected part of our veterinary training, and yet the area which underpins all our work. It ultimately determines not only how effectively we perform, but also the degree of professional satisfaction. We need to be both happy in our work and well financially stable before we can really begin to feel successful.

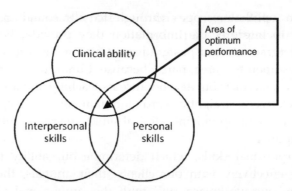

Figure 1.2 Achieving balance.

SUMMARY

Success in veterinary practice can mean different things to different people, but it should be based upon good clinical practice and sound business sense in order to be sustainable. This includes the application of best practice to our work, and the continual effort required to work towards quality patient and client care.

It has been necessary to consider just what 'quality' means within a veterinary context, since the definition of the term is not as obvious as it may first seem. The definition proposed by Moullin (2002) as 'meeting customer requirements and expectations at an acceptable price' does assume that the client always knows and desires what is in the best interests of their pet.

Other approaches to the issue of quality have taken a more client-centred approach, which is also highly relevant in the commercial world of veterinary practice. The work of Harr (2001) and David (1990) reminds us that we need to consider the client's experience that we offer as a whole, as well as the narrower issue of the quality of clinical care. It is only natural that as clinicians we are hung up on the latter, but it is far more frequently the broader client care issues that determine whether our customers return to us or not.

We have looked at the elements that characterize good practice from the point of view of the working environment, the individual character traits and the quality of output, although they are obviously all interlinked:

- The Hallmarks of Excellence that Neighbour (2005) proposed as key character traits are most closely related to a high level of performance as a practitioner.
- The Good Work Project (Gardner et al., 2006) examined the concept of moral identity within a professional context, and the four main areas that underpin it. Good Work is most likely to result when the required standards are clearly understood and the forces influencing them are well balanced.
- TQM as adapted for medical health care by Berwick (1989), and the ten steps required to achieve it within an organization.

Quality assurance is usually associated with manufacturing processes, but can actually be applied to a service industry as well. The three aspects of quality assurance outlined above can be visualized as influencing the three stages of an industrial process (Figure 1.3).

Quality comes with a cost, but the cost of offering poor quality care is usually a lot higher, both in terms of the cost of putting things right and the cost of lost business. We have examined why there may be a gap between the level of service that a client expects and that which they receive.

The question of what makes a veterinarian succeed in practice has no single answer. The concept of what comprises success is a personal one that needs to be identified before a path can be mapped out to achieve it. It is assisted by an examination of our own values and beliefs to establish why we have chosen to do what we do, and then identify our life goals. Only then can we develop a clear sense of mission to drive ourselves forward – these issues are developed in Chapter 3. We also have to find, or if it is within our power, create, a work culture that encourages good practice. But there has to be a market for what we would like to offer, whether it is as an employee or as a practice owner, or it will not be viable. So, we also need to consider what the consumer considers to be good veterinary practice, and find a practicable pathway that fits in as closely as possible with our own values.

RAW MATERIALS

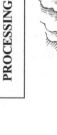

Veterinary practice is a service industry, and our 'raw materials' are the members of the practice team. Roger Neighbour's consideration of the Hallmarks of Excellence helps us to consider the desirable character traits for such work, and perhaps assists with the selection and training processes.

PROCESSING

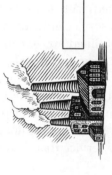

The 'factory' within the veterinary context is our working environment, not only in terms of the physical facilities, but also in terms of the practice ethos which helps to foster the development of Good Work, as considered by Howard Gardner and his colleagues at Harvard University.

OUTPUT

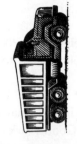

Our 'products' are the services that we deliver to our clients. Traditional quality control simply examines and attempts to maintain the quality of that product. Total quality management, as outlined by the Institute of Health Care Improvement, looks at all stages of the 'production process' to try and optimize the quality of care offered.

Figure 1.3 The path to good veterinary practice.

Finally, we have returned to the concept that over the long term, if we wish to strive for success we need to consider more than just the quality of clinical care that we provide, or even the overall client's experience that we offer. In order to thrive as a successful veterinarian throughout our career, we need to develop a harmonious balance of professional competencies that involves looking after ourselves and our team, as well as our clients.

If you just want to read one book...

Good Work: When Excellence and Ethics Meet by Professor Howard Gardner and his colleagues at Harvard Graduate School of Education makes interesting and stimulating reading. Some of the information, plus a lot of additional material, is available online at www.goodworkproject.org – and much of it can be downloaded free of charge.

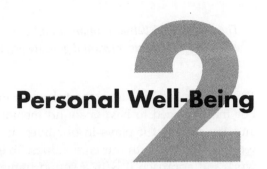

Personal Well-Being

The long period between infancy and our last years is a process of emerging from helplessness and gaining personal control. (Seligman, 1991)*

This book is all about a successful career in veterinary medicine. For that we need to have a sound mental attitude to our work and the part that it plays in our lives. It involves aligning our work in practice with our core values. To enable us to enjoy our work and approach it with a sound frame of mind, we need to find a happy balance between our work and the other things that are important to us. Otherwise we may be able to follow the rule books and achieve short-term success, but we will be doomed to long-term failure.

We are going to start by looking at human needs, particularly what is described as self-actualization, and then consider how the science of positive psychology may help us gain fulfilment from veterinary practice. We will examine the concept of flow, an absorption in our work that can enhance our sense of well-being if harnessed correctly. Emotional intelligence is a crucial skill that can also enhance our sense of well-being, as well as helping to develop the communication and leadership skills that are considered in later chapters.

A major barrier to our personal development is a lack of time, although sometimes we use it as an excuse for inactivity. We will examine some practical time management tips and consider how a lack of time and other pressures can lead to stress-related dysfunction in the workplace. Finally, we will examine how we can best find a harmonious balance between our work and the rest of our lives.

THE LUXURY OF SELF-ACTUALIZATION

Back in 1954, Abraham Maslow first identified what he described as the Hierarchy of Needs, starting with the most fundamental requirements at the base of the pyramid, such as food, shelter and

* This extract was published in *Learned Optimism*, Martin Seligman, Ph.D. Copyright © 2006 with permission from Random House, Inc.

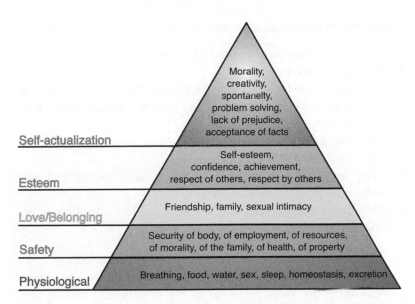

Self-actualization — Morality, creativity, spontaneity, problem solving, lack of prejudice, acceptance of facts

Esteem — Self-esteem, confidence, achievement, respect of others, respect by others

Love/Belonging — Friendship, family, sexual intimacy

Safety — Security of body, of employment, of resources, of morality, of the family, of health, of property

Physiological — Breathing, food, water, sex, sleep, homeostasis, excretion

Figure 2.1   Maslow's hierarchy of needs. Adapted from Maslow (1999).

sex. People will normally attempt to meet those needs before they move on to try and satisfying higher level of needs, such as companionship and competence, and then on to more sophisticated capacities such as generosity, forgiveness and self-discipline. Maslow felt that unfulfilled needs lower on the ladder would inhibit the person from climbing to the next step, illustrating it with the extreme example that someone dying of thirst quickly forgets their thirst when they have no oxygen. Those at the highest level of development are able to free themselves from some of the limitations of their biological heritage, exhibiting a sense of maturity and autonomy, developing unique abilities whilst also contributing to the well-being of their community (Figure 2.1).

To consider such development to be strictly hierarchical is obviously over-simplistic. For example, some highly creative people may pursue their craft even at the expense of the most basic necessities, but it is insightful to appreciate that as soon as a need is met, it ceases to become a motivator.

These concepts lead at their pinnacle to what Maslow describes as 'self-actualization'. He outlined the following characteristics shown by self-actualizing people:

- They are spontaneous in their ideas and actions.
- They are creative.
- They are interested in solving problems; this often includes the problems of others. Solving these problems is often a key focus in their lives.
- They feel a closeness to other people and generally appreciate life.
- They have a system of morality that is fully internalized and independent of external authority.
- They have discernment and are able to view all things in an objective manner.

In short, self-actualization is reaching one's fullest potential.

Those of us fortunate enough to be working in the veterinary profession in the Western world in the twenty-first century are likely to find all the more basic of our needs have been catered for. It is unlikely that we are going to be motivated by striving to meet physiological or physical safety needs, nor look to our professional lives to meet our needs for love and belonging, other than for friendship. But our professional careers may be critically important in meeting our needs for the various forms of esteem and provide an opportunity for fulfilling our more advanced needs.

Maslow specifically considered these traits in relation to a dedication to develop as a physician:

> *Self-actualization via being a physician means being a good physician, not a poor one. This ideal certainly is partly created by him, partly given to him by the culture, and partly discovered within himself...*

It is no coincidence that this bears some similarity to the concepts of Howard Gardner's Good Work Project as outlined in the previous chapter.

There can be little doubt that with a positive approach to our work, veterinary practice can provide an ideal pathway to what Maslow described as self-actualization.

MASLOW'S HIERARCHY – WHERE DO YOU STAND?

Look at Maslow's hierarchy and relate the needs to your own:

- Where do you think you stand within the pyramid?
- Are there needs that you feel are irrelevant to you?
- Have you fulfilled all the more basic needs or are there some that you are still striving to meet?
- Can you identify with the characteristics of self-actualized people that Maslow has identified?
- Are there other 'ideals' that you feel should be added to the list?
- Do you think that life in veterinary general practice gives you the space to develop those traits?
- Are there steps that you feel you could take to move closer to the ideals that you have identified?

POSITIVE PSYCHOLOGY

Since the end of the World War II, the science of psychology has been primarily focused upon dealing with mental illness, and its capacity to improve 'normal' lives has been largely overlooked. It is only as we have moved into the twenty-first century that the discipline of positive psychology has found its feet, particularly with the work of Barbara Fredrickson (2001), who demonstrated that positive affective experiences can have a long-lasting effect upon our personal growth and development in the following ways:

- Broadening our attention and thinking – when we experience positive emotions we are more likely to be creative, flexible and open-minded.
- Countering negative emotions – a deliberate experience of positive emotions can help to counteract the harmful psychological and physiological effects of negative ones.

- Enhancing our resilience and ability to cope with challenges. A positive approach fosters problem-focused coping, positive reappraisal of issues and infusing negative events with a positive meaning, which all facilitate our ability to cope with negative events.
- Building more permanent physical, intellectual, social and psychological resources that stand us in good stead over the longer term. Just as negative emotions can spiral downwards into a depressive state, positive ones can improve our longer term psychological well-being.

Sometimes, negative emotions do have their value, such as helping us to learn about ourselves. Wisdom is often gained from experiencing suffering and loss that are an intrinsic part of our existence. Yet, we do need to move on from traumatic experiences, and there are many techniques that positive psychology can offer to help enhance our positive emotions and so help us to cope better. For example:

- Physical and mental relaxation techniques such as progressive muscle relaxation, yoga and meditation exercises can help achieve a state of positive mindfulness.
- Training and support to help find meaning in our routine daily activities by reframing them in positive terms can help in general terms, but has also specifically been shown to enhance clinical problem solving in medical practitioners (Isen et al., 1991).
- Laughter and genuine smiling has been shown to be beneficial to those suffering bereavement (Keltner and Bonanno, 1997).

There is significant research that has shown that taking an optimistic stance to life can bring many benefits, such as:

- Less anxiety and depression
- Better adaptation to negative events such as serious illness
- The ability to learn positive lessons from negative events
- Better determination to continue with a task that proves challenging
- A tendency to partake in more health-promoting behaviours such as regular exercise and preventative medical care, and better long-term physical health

- Improved productivity in the workplace (Carver and Schier, 2002)

Admittedly, there are some occasions when pessimism can be advantageous, as optimism is associated with an underestimation of risks, and so optimists are more likely to partake in dangerous activities such as reckless driving. Pessimists may also be better prepared for calamitous events, even if optimists may be better able to recover from them. Perhaps it is preferable for the pilot of the plane you are flying into be a pessimist!

But customer service is paramount to the success of a veterinary practice, and a negative attitude is quickly transmitted to our clients. Upbeat moods at the interface with our customer base tend to influence our clients, so that they instinctively feel that our practice is a 'nice' place to visit – and they are more likely to respond positively as a result, which makes the whole process self-fulfilling; we start off with a positive frame of mind; our clients respond accordingly; and we end up getting more pleasure from the work that we do. The frame of mind of the leader will have a marked effect upon that of the team that are at work, so if the individual taking the leading role acts positively, its effect will be multiplied.

Overall, the ideal stance would seem to be one of positive realism, where the potential carelessness and unrealistic expectations of blind optimism is tempered by ensuring that wishful thinking is not allowed to cloud judgement.

The art, or many would argue, the science, of combating depression that results from a pessimistic stance has founded the now well-established school of cognitive therapy. Recent evidence has suggested that it is one of the most successful forms of psychotherapy, which aims at tackling the problem as it exists, rather than searching for underlying causes.

There is a significant body of work that asserts that whilst our attitudes may be founded upon strongly inherited tendencies, and early childhood experiences, it is possible to modify our behavioural stances. For further information on this topic, I would refer you to Martin Seligman's book, *Learned Optimism* (1991). But then, if you're a confirmed pessimist, you may not consider it worth trying.

TIP: FIVE STEPS TO LEARNED OPTIMISM

1. Learn to recognize the automatic thoughts that flit through your consciousness at the times that you feel worst.
2. Learn to dispute the automatic thoughts by marshalling contrary evidence.
3. Learn to make different explanations, or reattributions, and use them to dispute the automatic thoughts.
4. Learn how to distract yourself from depressing thoughts. This may mean putting off reflecting about your performance when you are actually under pressure, and learning to concentrate on carrying out the task in hand to the best of your abilities.
5. Learn to recognize and question the depression-sowing assumptions governing so much of what you do.

HAPPY VETERINARY PRACTICE

> *Happiness depends, as Nature shows,*
> *Less on exterior things than most suppose.*
> (William Cowper, 1782; 'Table Talk')

The word happiness sounds trite, so psychologists are much more prone to use the term 'subjective well-being' or never to miss an opportunity for an acronym, SWB. Trite or not, isn't it a major part of what we seek from our lives? Happiness as a construct involves more than just short-term happiness, or hedonistic pleasure, but also what Seligman (2002) describes as authentic happiness, which also involves the concept of 'self-validation'. Seligman rather neatly sums up the distinction as that between a 'pleasant life' and a 'good life'. It seems to be intrinsic to human nature that we will give up quite a lot of short-term pleasure in order to achieve what we consider to be worthwhile long-term goals, and it does seem as if this repays itself with a greater SWB in the long term.

It's no coincidence that this relates back to 'A look in the mirror' in the previous chapter, where we considered how a successful vocation can be summed up by a congruence between our values and the practice of our profession, so that we can metaphorically look ourselves in the mirror and say that we are satisfied with what we see. If we don't have a clearly identified value system, or if we find ourselves having to continually carry out work in a way that is contrary to our values, we are unlikely to end up happy in our work.

But is there anything we can do to influence the happiness that we experience in our lives? The zero-sum theory propounds that happiness is cyclical, with ups and downs, and anything we do to influence an 'up' will simply be counterbalanced by a lower 'down'. Adaptation theory predicts that happiness is influenced by major external events, be they lottery wins or serious accidents, but then returns quite quickly to a baseline level. Current thinking, as summarized by Seligman (2002), suggests that about 50% of SWB is genetically determined, objective life circumstances account for no more than 10% and the remaining 40% is under voluntary control – intentional activities that an individual can choose to engage in or not, to improve their SWB.

So, what are the life circumstances that are known to influence happiness? The results of psychological research do not always show up the answers we expect (Table 2.1).

Psychologist Ilona Boniwell also gives some fascinating facts about well-being:

- In three months the effect of promotion or being fired on well-being loses their impact.
- Winning the lottery often leaves people less happy.
- Real levels of income have risen dramatically in the prosperous nations over the past 50 years but SWB has remained flat.
- Recent changes in pay relate to job satisfaction but rates of pay do not.
- People in wealthier nations seem to have higher levels of happiness than those in poorer ones, but there are notable exceptions such as Brazil.
- Desiring wealth leaves one less happy.

So, what can you actively do, bearing in mind the principles of positive psychology, to influence the 40% of our SWB that is estimated to be amenable to such manipulation? I have taken

Table 2.1 Factors influencing our sense of well-being.

SWB is related to:	SWB is not particularly related to:
Optimism	Age (in fact older people are sometimes happier)
Extraversion	Physical attractiveness
Social connections especially close friendships	Money, once the basic needs are met
Being married	Gender (women are more often depressed but more often joyful)
Having engaging work	Education
Religion or spirituality (could be related to social connections)	Having children – especially under fives! But they may make your life more meaningful, and parents tend to live longer
Leisure	Moving to a sunnier climate
Good sleep and exercise	Crime prevention
Social class (through lifestyle differences and better coping strategies)	Housing
Subjective health (what you think about your health)	Objective health (what doctors think about your health)

After Boniwell (2006).

the liberty of paraphrasing some suggestions that Ilona Boniwell makes in her book, by putting them into a veterinary context. As you read through the list, think about what may work for you, and perhaps other activities that you might find preferable. Whatever you do, just the feeling that you are taking control of this part of your life is likely to have a beneficial effect upon your SWB – call it a placebo effect if you like!

- Focus beyond yourself and perform random acts of kindness – there are plenty of opportunities to do this in veterinary practice, but carry them out with a positive heart rather than feeling pressurized into them.
- Give priority and time to building on close relationships, especially with other long-term members of the practice team. It's not the quantity but the quality that counts.

- Treat yourself to a special day away from the practice, such as at a spa, and savour the experience without feeling guilty.
- Avoid the temptation to compare yourself negatively with those you perceive as being better off than yourself. Make a conscious effort to appreciate what you have.
- Look for new ways to carry out old procedures, to stop yourself from becoming jaded. Professionally, this ties in with a thirst to seek out new knowledge and applying it to your practice.
- Actively seek out challenges in carrying out even the most routine task supremely well. Even every vaccination visit is unique, and can be seen as an opportunity to strike up a relationship with a client and your patient, and thereby actively promote preventative health care.
- Reflect upon how you perform and give yourself credit for a case well handled, as well as taking forwards ideas on how to do it better. Focus upon the good things that veterinary practice can bring to your life, rather than harping upon the negatives.
- Try to take control of what you do and when you do it rather than just tagging along as the line of least resistance. Keep a sense of perspective about what really matters.
- Join up for some form of sports activity group that you find enjoyable. Both the physical and social activity will benefit your SWB and enhance your ability to do your job effectively. Additionally, this will help your sleep patterns, and ensuring you get the good quality of rest you need over a period of time is important.

TWO SHORT EXERCISES TO BOOST YOUR SENSE OF WELL-BEING

Most self-help exercises have not been proven to be effective, but these two little activities have been proven to have an effect, albeit transient, upon our SWB (Emmons and McCullough, 2003; Seligman, 2005):

1. Each day, for a fortnight, write down up to five things in your life that you are grateful or thankful for.
2. Write and deliver personally a letter of gratitude to someone who has been especially kind to you but who has never been properly thanked.

FLOW

Partaking in absorbing work and hobbies is another behaviour that may enhance our SWB, and it is one that pretty much comes with the job. The state described as 'flow' is when we become totally focused upon such an activity and lose all sense of the passage time, or even emotion. The state has been extensively re-searched by Mihaly Csikszentmihalyi (1992), who discovered that it occurs only under certain conditions – the task in hand needs to challenge our skills, yet we need to be just about capable of them, so that we do not become frustrated. Many activities apart from our work are conducive to flow, such as sports, dancing, art, sex, socializing and reading.

I'm sure that most of us have experienced the satisfaction of coming to the end of a demanding morning's operating list, where everyone has worked together as a team and what seemed daunt-ing before it began seemed to be over in a flash. Csikszentmihalyi identified certain characteristics of the experience:

- Clarity of goals and an immediate feedback of performance.
- The activities are intrinsically rewarding.
- Complete concentration on the issue in hand with no time for distraction by other issues.
- Actions and awareness are merged – so a surgeon may get the sensation that he or she actually becomes at one with his or her instruments, and the activity almost effortless despite its complexity.
- Losing an awareness of oneself – although paradoxically one's sense of self-awareness may increase after the activity ceases.
- Sense of control over what one is doing, with complete self-confidence.

- Transformation of time, so that usually it passes much faster than expected.

Not everything that brings us short-term pleasure is likely to result in a state of flow, particularly if participation is passive and undemanding – watching television is a prime example of such an activity, which is likely to result in a more apathetic response rather than a positive one.

So, is flow necessarily a positive experience? It can have a negative impact, where people become addicted to the stimulation to the point where it disrupts their normal lives. As Mihaly Csikszentmihalyi says:

'The flow experience, like everything else, is not "good" in an absolute sense. It is good only in that it has the potential to make life more rich, intense and meaningful; it is good because it increases the strengths and complexity of the self. But whether the consequence of any instance of flow in good in a larger sense needs to be discussed and evaluated in terms of more inclusive social criteria'. The question regarding flow is not only how we can make it happen, but also how we can manage it: using it to enhance life; yet being able to let go when necessary.

Flow can be an introverted experience, but it can also be shared by a group working together, when it can act as an extremely strong bonding and motivating force. It is worth encouraging in a practice, as the excitement and elation of completing a job well done is multiplied when it is accompanied by a heightened sense of camaraderie. Those of us who enjoy surgery will recognize the 'buzz' that working through a demanding operating list or a really busy period of consulting effectively and efficiently as a team can bring. When it occurs, it should be recognized and celebrated to help practice team building.

EMOTIONAL INTELLIGENCE

Recognizing our state of mind when in flow is just one aspect of emotional intelligence (EI), popularized by Daniel Goleman in his landmark book (1995). It refers to the capacity to recognize and manage our own emotions and the emotions of others with whom we interact. This is a skill that would logically seem to be important for our personal development, but may also be vitally important to successful interactions with our clients and with other members of our clinical team. The concept is being widely encouraged in many organizational contexts, particularly education, but there has been very little work reviewing its relevance to health care in general, and none relating to veterinary practice. Yvonne Birks (2007) reviewed the medical literature on the relationship between EI and patient-centred health care. It was not surprising that within a working environment where so much depends upon the relationship between the clinician and the patient, she was able to identify many potential areas of benefit.

There are four major facets of EI that need to be developed:

1. Perceiving emotions – the ability to read emotional messages, both verbal and non-verbal, which enables one to understand issues from the perspective of our clients and our colleagues and so act more empathetically.
2. Using emotions to facilitate thinking – if we recognize how emotions affect our thinking, we can utilize them to assist our problem-solving, reasoning and creative abilities.
3. Understanding emotions – we don't just need to recognize emotions, we need to be able to understand what is behind them, both in ourselves and in those with whom we come into contact. Although we may be experiencing those emotions ourselves, our conscious mind is often blissfully unaware of just why we are feeling as we are. Many of the decisions that our clients make about treatment options will be based upon emotions rather than pure logic. This is particularly true in the companion animal field, where the bond is usually almost entirely an emotional one, but even in production animal practice, conflicting emotions can play a significant role in the decisions that are taken.
4. Managing emotions – emotional management is not about eliminating emotions from our daily lives and interactions, but learning how to recognize them and then how to deal with

them. We can learn how to take positive steps to make ourselves feel better when we are down, and as we become more expert practitioners, we can learn how help our clients to deal with their emotions as well.

These competences can also be thought of as being either internal or external (Figure 2.2).

Empathy is obviously a central concept to EI, and it is important to understand what it means; it is different to sympathy, which implies sharing other people's feelings. It involves sensing other people's emotions, understanding their significance, and taking an active interest in their concerns – very different from adopting everyone else's feelings as our own and trying to please everyone. Empathy is essential to social effectiveness in our working lives and so maintains cohesive teamwork. Empathetic behaviour involves:

- Recognizing and taking into account the needs of clients, customers and subordinates.
- Being approachable so that people feel they want to hear what they have to say.
- Listening carefully to what they are told and responding appropriately.
- Being attuned to subtleties of body language and the emotional message beneath the words.

There are many techniques that have been used to help enhance our emotional management, the most obvious being that of consciously developing an improved awareness of our own emotions, and of those around us. The website http://www. eiconsortium.org/provides a great deal of background research and helpful information on the subject, including 22 guidelines for Best Practice for promoting EI in the workplace.

TIME MANAGEMENT

First, the bad news: research has shown that none of the many time training courses are likely to have any long-term effect upon

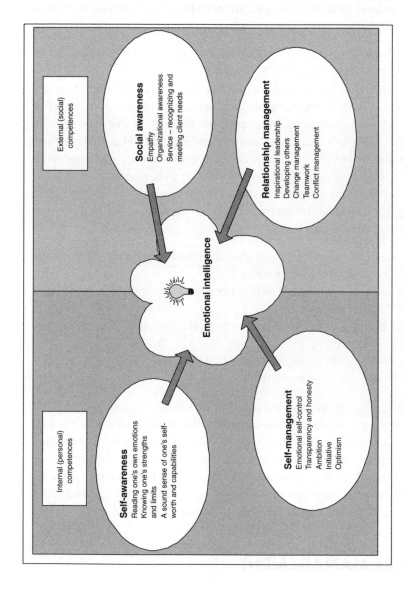

Figure 2.2 The four main aspects of emotional intelligence.

Internal (personal) competences

External (social) competences

Self-awareness
Reading one's own emotions
Knowing one's strengths and limits
A sound sense of one's self-worth and capabilities

Social awareness
Empathy
Organizational awareness
Service – recognizing and meeting client needs

Self-management
Emotional self-control
Transparency and honesty
Ambition
Initiative
Optimism

Relationship management
Inspirational leadership
Developing others
Change management
Teamwork
Conflict management

Emotional intelligence

the way you manage your time (Macan, 1996), which makes them a waste of time. The best I can hope to do is to stimulate you to think about how you utilize this precious commodity so that you yourself gain some insight as to where you could use it more effectively.

PRACTICAL TIME MANAGEMENT TIPS

- Don't confuse a lack of time with a lack of motivation. If you want to do something badly enough, you will find the time to do it.
- We often procrastinate about doing things, and they get put to the bottom of the pile due to 'lack of time', but there are usually other reasons why we are not doing them. Often it is because we are uneasy about the task, or unclear about what is required of us, or simply because we find it unpleasant. If it is because the task seems overwhelming, splitting it up into smaller, more manageable chunks will help.
- We all have a tendency to deal with urgent tasks first, regardless of how important they are. Recognize that some tasks are important but not urgent, and if necessary, put aside those that are pressing but not important. Many of these pressing but unimportant tasks will evaporate if ignored as they are superseded by developments.
- The sense that unfinished tasks are building up results in a feeling of lack of control and therefore work-related stress. It helps to compile a timeline over a manageable period of say, two months, and map out the tasks that need to be completed at a specific time and those that have no specific time limit. They can then be matched to the time available and prioritized accordingly. Ticking one off the list as it is completed brings its own pleasure. Mapping them out does not create more time, but gets them out of our heads and so helps stop us tossing and turning at night about them.
- Discard items that have been in your in-tray or on your To-Do list for longer than a month, unless you have clearly identified them as long-term aims. If they were that important, you would have been forced to do them before.

- Personal organizer software such as Outlook has become very sophisticated, and can be synchronized with hand-held PDAs that are increasingly merging with mobile telephones. These can be an excellent means of creating daily 'To-Do' lists and reminding us of tasks that need to be done, but we need to use them selectively so that we do not become slaves to our PDAs. Many practice management systems now have diaries and reminders build it.
- Don't be afraid to say 'No' when asked to do something. Our decision should be based upon how highly you would prioritize the task amongst the others that you have to do, and you should avoid agreeing to do something simply out of guilt, or to get someone off your back.

There is a big paradox between our perception of free time and the reality. Social scientists tell us that on average, since 1965, we have gained between five and seven more free hours per week. On average people estimate they have less than 20 hours of free time a week, but that is actually half of what they actually have. The leisure time that we do have is characterized by an increase in passive leisure and an intensification of the time devoted to active leisure – in other words, we spend more than 14 hours a week in front of our TV screens, eating up all of the extra leisure time we have earned. We now spend less time on the pastimes we tend to find most pleasurable such as socializing and outdoor activities. When we do engage in active leisure, we cram a larger number of activities into a shorter space of time, leading to feelings of fragmentation and time strain.

The key to time management is primarily not how to organize our lives to give ourselves more leisure time, but how to organize our time so that it best contributes to our well-being. More information on information management in general can be found in Chapter 5.

AN EXERCISE IN TIME MANAGEMENT

Keep a diary for a fairly typical week of how you spend your time throughout each day. Then categorize it so that you get an overview of how you use your time. A handy software tool called tiyga (pronounced 'tiger') can be downloaded free of charge on a trial basis to help you do that at www.tiyga.com.

- Are you surprised by how your time was allocated?
- How effectively do you consider you have used your time?
- Were there things that you did that would have been better delegated?
- Were there things you did that you would have been better off not doing at all?
- Are there things that you did that you feel could have been spent more usefully?
- Were there things that you did not do that needed doing?
- If so, was a lack of time the reason for not doing them, and could you have dealt with that more effectively?
- What do you feel about the overall work/life balance (WLB) during that week?
- Are there any actions within your influence that you could take to move closer to your ideal?

STRESS

Time pressure is a common cause of stress, which is a physiological response to any of a wide variety of challenges. As such, it can be a perfectly normal and healthy reaction, but we tend to think of stress as universally bad. When the demands exceed the personal and social resources that we are able to mobilize, we experience a loss of control and negative emotions. So, here is the bad news according to the analysis of a questionnaire sent out by David Bartram and his colleagues (2009) to over 3000 veterinarians in the UK. Compared to the general population they suffer from:

- Higher levels of anxiety and depressive symptoms
- Higher 12-month prevalence of suicidal thoughts (21.3%)
- Less favourable psychosocial work characteristics, especially in regard to demands and managerial support
- Lower levels of positive mental well-being
- Higher levels of negative work–home interaction

Focus groups of veterinarians found that clinicians identified the top three causes of stress as:

- The possibility of complaints and litigation
- Unexpected clinical outcomes
- After hours on-call duties

The top five sources of job satisfaction were:

- Good clinical outcomes
- Relationships with colleagues
- Intellectual challenge
- Client satisfaction
- Relationships with clients

Peter Warr (2007) reviewed the research regarding factors that influence happiness at work, and concluded that a feeling of lack of control over our working environment contributes strongly to the sense of despair that results in long-term stress and sometimes eventually meltdown.

Paradoxically, we spend a big chunk of our time trying to minimize stress, and a whole lot more finding ways of putting it back – be it by competitive sports, gambling, action and horror movies or extramarital affairs. It does seem that we have some innate desire to be stressed, and if channelled in the right directions a moderate degree of stress is part and parcel of the 'normal' life experience.

Stress is not an illness, but when excessive it can certainly trigger pathological changes that may well need professional help to tackle. But what techniques can we use ourselves to deal with stress?

David Bartram and Dianne Gardner (2008) recommend that the first step in dealing with work-related stress is to identify the individual stressors causing the problem. For example, stress due to complex issues such as 'staff relationships' or 'difficult clients' can only be dealt with if they are broken down into specific stressors which can then be considered individually, and the best method of coping selected.

These really boil down to just two methods: problem-focused coping and emotion-focused coping. A third option, avoidance coping, involves blocking it out of our minds with the help of distractions such as drugs, alcohol, sex, or even work, but is only a very short-term remedy.

Problem-focused coping is the rational process of identifying the causes of the stress and finding solutions to remove them. It's what generally comes naturally to veterinarians because of our professional selection and training, and it's what most of this chapter has been about.

That is all good and well when we can control the causes of the stress, but when we cannot (for example, when we suffer a bereavement), we need to turn to emotion-focused coping. This might include techniques such as seeking social support, self-control over one's own emotional reactions, and denial – trying to ignore the problem in the hope that it will go away. Whilst this may seem obvious, research has shown that veterinary students in an Australian veterinary school often did not consistently employ a range of effective coping strategies (Williams et al., 2005), and there is little to suggest that practicing veterinarians are any better at dealing with it.

Where active problem-focused coping is available as an option, it is more likely to bring long-term positive results than emotion-focused coping, but veterinarians may well continue to struggle to find a solution to a problem way past the point that that strategy is still viable.

TIP: EMOTION-FOCUSED STRATEGIES THAT MAY HELP COPE WITH STRESS

- Use humour to lighten a situation. Try and see the funny side of things.
- Reframe the situation in terms of importance and long-term impact, which may help put it into perspective.
- Confide in someone else. A problem shared can be a problem halved.
- Seek professional emotional support when appropriate. Ironically, professionals such as veterinarians often leave this too late.

- Try and be accepting of the situation rather than struggling against it. Feeling hard done by will only make matters worse. All things must pass.
- Divert your attention by working on another absorbing task.
- Concentrate on pleasant thoughts, rather than harping on negative ones. When you get a difficult client, make a conscious effort to remember all the pleasant ones. I keep a file with all my 'Thank you' letters to turn to when things get really rough.
- Engage in physical exercise. Yoga relaxes the mind as well as the body.
- Try and see the situation from a different perspective, particularly looking for positive benefits that might come from it, even if it is just learning how to deal with adversity.
- Turn the problem over to a higher authority to deal with it, such as the practice manager or senior partner. Don't get stressed about issues that are actually not your problem or that you don't have the authority to deal with.
- Spend time with your pets. They can be great for reducing stress.
- Compare yourself to others who are facing even more challenging situations – you will always be able to find someone worse off than you.
- Write down your thoughts and feelings. This might help you to find a solution to the problem, but if not, it will help to get it off your chest and reduce the need to churn the thoughts over in your mind.

ACHIEVING BALANCE

Feeling out of control of our own lives can have a significant negative effect upon our physical and psychological health via the stress response (Rodin, 1986).

One of the themes that runs through this book is the need to clarify the values that are important to you and then set achievable goals to allow you to advance your career in a way that fits in with those core values. By being proactive, rather than just reacting to outside forces that come your way, you can take control of your life. It is the feeling of being 'out of control' that is a major contributor to work-related stress and professional burn-out. But our life is more than just our work. Factors that are likely to be important include:

1. Career
2. Financial well-being
3. Physical health
4. Family and friends
5. Personal relationships and love
6. Personal development
7. Hobbies and social life
8. Our immediate environment

Each of us will have different priorities, and it is worth taking time to consider how important each of these areas is to you, which will help you to find a balance between your paid employment and your life outside of your career. Achieving a healthy WLB is all about making the right amount of time in your life in proportion to their importance to ourselves, taking steps towards ensuring that we drive our career forwards rather than our careers taking control of our lives. Just as with quality improvement, this is usually not achievable in one large leap, but rather in a series of small steps. Providing that we have a clear idea in our mind about where we are heading, small and steady steps will usually provide a safer journey towards reaching our ultimate goal, rather than large and potentially uncoordinated leaps.

In a survey carried out by the SPVS Masters Group (2003) responded to by over 1000 veterinarians in the UK, one question asked them to rank how important they felt a whole range of issues were in terms of how they were likely to impact upon their work in the future. Interestingly, changes to WLB legislation obtained the lowest score of all the factors, with only about 50% of practitioners rating it as likely to be very important or important and about 20% not even being aware of it as an issue.

Yet the evidence suggests that WLB issues are becoming increasingly important, with whole rafts of legislation being introduced in most Western countries to enhance the rights of workers and to try and reduce work-related stress. Getting it right benefits the practice as well as each individual within it, because it has been shown to:

- Increase productivity
- Improve recruitment and retention
- Lower rates of absenteeism
- Reduce overheads
- Improve customer experience
- Provide a more motivated, satisfied and equitable workforce

It is an example where the concerns of the profession seem to be out of tune with where our priorities ought best to lie, and with the concerns of society as a whole.

CHECK YOUR OWN WLB

Photocopy the 'Wheel of Life' diagram below, and then rate your own scores for each area of your life. You can adapt the axes if you feel there are other headings that would be more relevant to you, or you easily find computerized versions by entering the term into Google. Some wheels take a very general overview of your life, others have axes that relate to more specific areas. For example, a wheel that focused upon your health may have spokes relating to issues such as fitness, diet, weight, alcohol intake etc. Once you have built up your wheel and added your scores, join the dots you have made (Figure 2.3).

Look at the pattern that you have produced and see how well balanced you feel your life is. It should ideally be a big, round wheel, and if it is very uneven it indicates you have significant imbalances in your life. If this is the case, start to work out an action plan to achieve a better equilibrium in small, achievable steps. Repeat the exercise regularly to look for changes.

SUMMARY

In order to practice effectively we need to start with a good grounding of who we are, what we want to be, and how we want

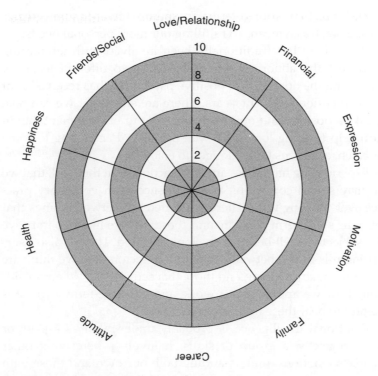

Figure 2.3   Wheel of life.

to get there. We can start with an understanding of the different levels of 'needs' that motivate us. As veterinarians, this is generally going to be more than to meet our basic physiological and security requirements, and we are likely to look to our work to provide esteem in its various forms and as we develop further. We can strive towards what Maslow described as self-actualization, or our full potential, although it is debatable as to whether we can actually reach it or whether it is a moving goal-post. Our path may be through personal development, or ultimately through serving some greater good. It's important to appreciate that whereas a philosophical or religious viewpoint may take a moral stance, the psychological basis for striving to benefit those other than ourselves is more pragmatic: we simply seem to be most satisfied in the long term when we do so. There is ample scope for us to use our veterinary expertise towards some greater good as well as a means to fulfilling our more personal needs.

Psychology has traditionally been involved with attempting to correct the abnormal, but it has a lot to offer in terms of enhancing the normal, and positive psychology has received a lot more attention in recent years. There are steps that we can take to take a positive and optimistic view of our environment that in turn help to bring long-term well-being, and according to some research, allows us to live longer to enjoy it.

Experiencing happiness and satisfaction from the work that we do may sound corny, but its key to success in veterinary practice over the long term. There is a difference between things that bring us short-term pleasure and those that are likely to improve our subjective well-being over a longer period. There is also a surprising mis-match between the external factors that we think are going to make us happy, and those that actually do. When considering how we approach our work, and our long-term goals, it is helpful to bear these findings in mind.

Emotional Intelligence is probably under-rated as a skill, or more correctly, a group of skills. It involves perceiving other people's emotions, understanding both our own and those with whom we interact, using that understanding to facilitate our reasoning, and managing emotions. By developing these skills, it can help us to plan and to run our own lives, as well as helping us in our interactions with our clients and the practice team, and thus improve our quality of practice.

We can often organize what we do more efficiently, and a lack of time in absolute terms is not the most common reason for us feeling under pressure. We have looked at steps that we can take to get a handle on the various demands, so that we feel more in control of our lives and consequently less troubled. But we should also consider whether we use our leisure time to obtain the maximum enhancement of our well-being. If we are convinced that watching television is the best way to spend a large proportion of it, that is fine, but we should make that decision as an active one rather than as the path of least resistance.

It would be great if we could positively influence all the factors in our working and personal environments in order to eliminate stress, but life just isn't like that. In fact, our behaviour suggests that up to a point we actively seek out stress. When factors beyond our control cause unacceptable levels the only effective antidote is emotion-focused coping. It seems likely that veterinarians are relatively poor at switching from problem-focused to emotion-focused coping, and this could account for the high levels of suicide within the profession. It is important for us to develop the EI to recognize and deal with such issues, and to seek professional help when appropriate.

The theme of balance is a very important one throughout this book, and I have ended the chapter with a discussion of the 'bigger picture' of where our work should fit into our lives. There is no right answer to fit everyone, but there are techniques that we can use to evaluate our various priorities and so set goals that will help us to work towards a situation where we are likely to find harmony and thus improved subjective well being.

If you just want to read one book...

I would strongly recommend Illona Boniwell's little handbook that is a really superb summary of positive psychology and all that it entails.
Boniwell, I. (2006). *Positive Psychology in a Nutshell*. London: PWBC.

Beliefs, Values, Goals and Motivation

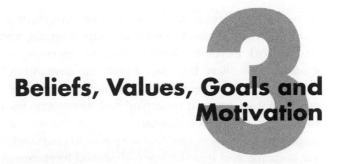

The pursuit of excellence calls for a clear vision, a clear sense of mission, and a clearing away of obstacles. (Neighbour, 2005)*

The previous chapter considered our attitudes to our work, our awareness of our own and other people's emotions, and how our work can effectively fit into the 'bigger picture' of our lives. Before we move on to consider some more practical aspects of how we can strive towards success, I want to take a little more time to consider our beliefs and values that underpin our work. Most

* This extract was published in *The Inner Apprentice*, second edition, Roger Neighbour. Oxford: Radcliffe Publishing. © 2005 Roger Neighbour. Reproduced with the permission of the copyright holder.

of us initially decide to follow a career in veterinary medicine out of a desire to work with and 'help' animals, and then have had to work incredibly hard to get into veterinary school and to graduate. We were then faced with the demands of veterinary practice, which challenge even the most confident new graduate, and before we know it we are up and running on the treadmill of life as a practicing veterinarian.

At some stage it is vital that we pause to take stock of where we are heading, and this chapter is designed to encourage reflection about just what being a veterinary professional actually means, and the pathway that each of us wishes to follow within that profession. Once we have a clear picture of our personal goals, we can then begin to consider how we can best fulfil our objectives.

BELIEFS AND VALUES

Shaping strategic success requires organizations to recognize and articulate those values that drive its decisions and to disseminate those values throughout the organization. (Pfeiffer et al., 1989)

Those words accurately capture the essence of what distinguishes many successful organizations from those that fail to prosper, but the same sentiment can be applied to us as individuals. It may seem strange to say that we need to articulate our values – if we own them, surely we know what they are? Yet we very rarely take a pause from the demands of our professional lives to think about the beliefs and values that should guide how we act. Each of us benefits from taking time to reflect upon how our beliefs and values apply to our work, and how closely we can match up what we feel in intrinsically important with the reality of what we actually do. But let's start by considering what those two terms actually mean.

Beliefs can be described as broad, simplistic summaries of what we have learned during our formative years – working hypotheses. Very often, our beliefs may be based upon false premises and perceptions, yet we often fail to re-evaluate them in the light of our day-to-day experiences. For example, our parents may have always treated one of our siblings as the beauty of the family, and subliminally led us to believe that we are physically unattractive. That belief may stay with us throughout our lives, even though we may have been attractive all along, or an ugly duckling that has developed into a veritable swan. Our attitude to our patients will be strongly influenced by our beliefs. For example, we may believe that animals have been put on earth to serve humankind; we may believe in the theory of evolution and that animals are sentient beings whose welfare we need to consider when impinge upon them; or we may believe that all animals, including humans, have fundamental rights that we are morally obliged to respect.

In everyday transactions, **values** are more in evidence than beliefs. They are a form of mental architecture that help to inform our decision making so that it accords with what we believe, and to provide a sense of consistency and purpose when we consider our options. They are effectively beliefs chopped down to size for application at single decision points, to be applied to desirable states or modes of conduct, whereas beliefs are the total condensation of what our experiences have taught us so far. For example, whatever your belief about the place of animals in the world, one of your core values may be to ensure as best as you can the welfare of animals that are entrusted into your care. Many of our beliefs and values have been handed down 'en bloc' by those who have influenced us in our formative years, but they will usually evolve as we develop. Just occasionally, we may experience very significant transformations in our belief and corresponding value systems, which are likely to have a considerable impact upon the way in which we run our lives.

Modern society no longer offers us a rigid set of values in the way that it used to, and we now are much more open to the concept that others may have values that are different to ours, and with that ours become, to some extent, arbitrary. Shwartz (1994) proposed ten motivationally distinct values that he found to be common to all cultures:

• Power – social status and prestige. Control or dominance over people or resources

- Achievement – personal success through the demonstration of competence
- Hedonism – pleasure and sensuous gratification for ourselves
- Stimulation – excitement, novelty and challenge in our lives
- Self-direction – independent thought and action
- Universalism – understanding, appreciation and tolerance, and protection for the welfare of all people and nature (particularly animals in our instance)
- Benevolence – preservation and enhancement of the welfare of people with whom we are in frequent contact
- Tradition – respect, commitment and acceptance of the customs and ideas that traditional culture or religion provide
- Conformity – restraint of actions and inclinations likely to upset and harm others or violate social expectations or norms
- Security – safety, harmony and stability of society, of relationships and of ourselves

To some extent, these groups of values are potentially in conflict with each other. For example, conformity and tradition are conservative values that may be diametrically opposed to hedonism, stimulation and self-direction. Similarly, the self-transcendental values of universalism and benevolence may conflict with the self-enhancement required for power and achievement. Prioritizing and reconciling these different types of values is one of the major challenges facing our societies at large, and ourselves as individuals functioning within those frameworks.

When there is a conflict between what we do and what our values lead us to think we should be doing, we may actively change our values. Alternatively, we may be able to compartmentalize them, accepting different values in different circumstances. Some would call that hypocrisy, but others see these value conflicts as an inevitable part of our complex human psyches, and an important part of the learning process. By constantly challenging and re-evaluating our values, we can adapt them and find an optimum balance between our underlying beliefs and the behavioural options that face us when we are called upon to make decisions.

Success in veterinary practice depends upon a matching of personal and professional values with those required of the job. Serious mismatches may be glossed over or ignored for a time, but eventually they will rise to the surface and cause at best, suboptimal performance, and at worst, complete dysfunction and breakdown. The corollary of this is that a clear idea of what our values actually are does not only enable us to make decisions effectively, it also allows us to create goals for ourselves: if we value things highly enough, we don't just wait for them to happen: we actively seek them out. Opportunities are not just seized, they can be created. When values obtain the motivational energy to make things happen, and carve out a path towards our personal goals in a sustained and coordinated way, they lead to what can best be described as a mission.

Living to one's values leads to integrity, and integrity enables transparency, an authentic openness to others about one's feelings, beliefs and actions. Integrity leads to trust, which is a vital quality within any organization.

Identifying Your Own Value Set

Review the universal list of values as proposed by Schwartz above, and consider each area in more detail:

- What does it mean to you?
- How important is it to you?
- How closely are you able to follow each value in your life?
- How much effort do you think it is worth expending in trying to move towards your ideal?
- Are there any missing values that you would like to add to your own personal list?

Carried out thoroughly, this is a formidable mind exercise. If you write down your conclusions, you can refer back to them after a period of time, and audit how your own values have changed, and whether you have been able to constructively modify your own behaviour in any way.

PROFESSIONALISM

Being a professional means that an individual conforms to a set of values that are in some way different to those of the community at large. It's one of those terms whose meaning is commonly understood yet is notoriously difficult to pin down, but most would agree with the truism that professional behaviour is integral to good veterinary practice.

A summit of British medical organizations (Smith, 1994) came up with the following behaviours that should epitomize a medical professional:

- Caring
- Integrity
- Competence
- Confidentiality
- Responsibility
- Advocacy

Sue Shuttleworth (2006) considered the meaning of professionalism within a veterinary context as part of her Doctoral thesis, and concluded that it meant:

- Believing passionately in what you do
- Critically reflecting on the work you carry out in relation to personal, peer and eminence-based standards and values
- Learning from your experiences in an ongoing and positive way
- Caring about your clients and their animals, your practice team and your career
- Doing what you consider is the professional thing to do in any circumstances

Considering Professionalism

Write down your responses to the following questions:

- As a professional I enjoy a privileged position. What core values do I hold that justify society entrusting me with power and prestige?

- Which professionals do I respect the most, and why? (This should include other veterinarians, but not necessarily exclude those from outside.)

PROFESSIONAL ETHICS

Ethics are the 'rules of conduct' which we feel should govern our actions, or within this context, the rules to which we feel that members of the veterinary profession should adhere. Morality describes the degree to which we are able to put those ethical rules into effect. When we agree to become a member of the veterinary profession, we agree to accept an ethical code of conduct, that may be implicit, or more commonly explicitly described in a code.

Problems may arise when either the code of conduct that governs our professional behaviour differs with our own personal values, or we are faced with particular circumstances where our personal values may be brought into conflict with our professional duty. If you think such issues are rare in practice, you are failing to recognize them when they occur. These matters do not just crop up on an occasional basis, but affect the day-to-day manner in which we carry out our work. For example, every time we recommend a course of treatment, we face a potential conflict of interest between benefit to the patient, the cost to the owner and the benefit to the practice from the financial profit generated. A conflict of interest is a *condition* and not a *behaviour* – in other words, it exists whether we allow it to influence our behaviour or not, and so needs to be overtly recognized.

Ethical issues are rarely matters of clearly right or wrong. Later on in the book, we look at the nature of knowledge, and also discover how developing our emotional intelligence and reflective practice skills helps us to appreciate that there are different ways of interpreting most of these issues. That does not mean that we necessarily have to agree with those views, but by understanding their nature, we can deal with their consequences more effectively.

A good starting point for any consideration of veterinary ethics are the four guiding principles developed within the medical context by Beauchamp and Childress (2001). In no particular order they are:

- Respect for autonomy (people's right to make their own decisions)
- Beneficence (providing a net benefit)
- Non-maleficence (doing no harm)
- Justice (acting fairly)

These four principles can be used to analyse any ethical dilemma and to help identify the best way forward.

Veterinary welfare and ethics has become a major branch of veterinary science in its own right, and there are excellent books that have been written on the subject. It is not within the scope of this book to go into individual ethical dilemmas that face veterinarians in practice, but hopefully the cognitive skills that this book will help to provide at least some of the tools that are required to deal with such issues.

An Exercise in Ethics

Think about an ethical dilemma that has faced you in your work. Examples might include being asked to carry out a course of action by an owner that conflicts with what you consider to be right, or where outside pressures such as finances may impinge upon the course of clinical action that you might take.

- Write down the issues as you see them, but from the point of view of each of the parties involved.
- Write down what you consider to be your core values that relate to that issue and any conflicts that may have arisen.
- Try and analyse the various options in terms of the four guiding principles outlined above.
- Reflect upon how this might affect the actions that you might take in similar circumstances in the future.

LIFE GOALS

Pay the right kind of attention to the here and now, and the rest will follow. (Neighbour, 2005)

Goals are thoughts about desired states or outcomes that we would like to achieve, that are based upon our values. Life goals are specific motivational objectives by which we live our lives. They are different to needs because they are formulated at the conscious level, and differ from short-term goals because they guide the way we run our lives for an extended duration.

If this were a book about running a good veterinary practice, it would launch straight into a section about goal setting, because it is undeniable that success in business depends upon striving towards a clearly spelt-out mission by means of well-defined goals based on sound values. But it's about success in our careers, and that can mean many different things. Not everyone wants to be a business entrepreneur, or even take on the responsibilities involved in partnership. Your priorities may be focused around advancing your clinical skills, mentoring other professionals, or perhaps centred around the provision of charitable assistance. More likely, it will involve a combination of different areas, but you may afford each a different level of priority.

It is worth mentioning that the Buddhist viewpoint takes this further and believes that all life's suffering stems from attachment to goals, and that we should concentrate on awareness of the here and now rather than continually striving for something new. Looking at things from that viewpoint, capitalism depends upon the attachment to goals in order to generate a continual requirement for further production to meet the demand for new acquisitions. A sobering thought, and even if it does not have you reaching for your saffron robes, it should again prompt you to think very carefully about your parameters for success before you start striving to reach them. Even a somewhat puzzled Sigmund Freud had to admit:

> People occasionally fall ill precisely because a deeply rooted and long-cherished wish has come to fulfillment. It seems as though they could not endure their bliss.

There is something about human nature that drives us to extreme lengths to realize an ambition, and yet undervalue it once we have achieved it. Many of us are so goal-orientated that we never really stop to appreciate what we have. The ability to overcome formidable obstacles to reach our goals is widely valued in Western society: the ability to appreciate what we already have is valued less.

Very often it is the *process* of pursuing life goals that brings us happiness, rather than their realization. This is the simple fact that can come as a major blow to someone who manages to achieve their life goals, suddenly realizing that they are left with nothing further for which to strive. We need to consider this very carefully when formulating our life goals, and consider from the outset whether we are happy to continually re-set our goals so that we always have new ones to chase, or whether we feel able to achieve true happiness when we reach them. Executive coaching has sprung up as a very viable profession to help high-fliers to clarify their objectives, and to try and equate achievement with satisfaction, as the two so often fail to go hand in hand.

Erich Fromm (1976) made a distinction between a 'having' orientation and a 'being' orientation, with the former focused around accumulating wealth and status and the latter about self-actualization. He discovered that people with 'being' orientated life goals were on average happier than those seeking fame and fortune. However, later research (Oishi et al., 1999) has suggested that it is not so much the content of the life goals themselves that determines our happiness, but the congruence between the values that a person holds, and their goals. It might seem that everyone's goals fit in with their values, but there are many outside influences that may influence the goals that we seek. It seems that quite often we do not stop to think how closely they match our values before chasing after them and eventually becoming disillusioned. Psychologists tell us that life satisfaction is simply a congruence between the present and an ideal situation, both of which are a reflection of each person's own subjective appreciation of life (Diener, 1984).

Lyuborminsky (2001) discovered that well-being is enhanced when people pursue goals which are:

- Feasible, realistic and attainable
- Those they are already making progress towards

- Personally meaningful and 'owned' by us rather than imposed upon us
- Those to which people feel highly committed
- Concerned with community, intimacy and growth
- Self-concordant and congruent with people's motives and needs
- Valued by one's culture
- Not conflicting with each other

So, why do we so often fail to pursue them effectively? Ford and Nichols (1991) propose three convincing reasons:

1. We often end up pursuing short-term goals that are more urgent but less important than our long-term ones, because they demand our immediate attention. We need to deal with urgent matters as they arise, but ensure that we have protected time to attend to our long-term priorities.
2. Most of us have an inbuilt fear of failure, so sometimes we do not wholeheartedly set out to reach our life goals, even though we know they are important.
3. Worthwhile goals usually require perseverance, and we may run out of energy and give up before we have achieved them.

The happiness that achieving goals may bring to us partly depends upon our own intrinsic nature, but also upon the type of goals that we select. Seligman (2002) describes three types of goals and the happiness that each is likely to bring:

- **Positive emotion** – the pleasant life. In the past tense this would involve states such as contentment, satisfaction, serenity and pride. Looking into the future they would include hope, optimism, faith and trust. In the 'now' this involves sensations of pleasure such as leisure, sex, rest or play. They all result in pleasant feelings, that can make people feel more energetic, and bring a more positive attitude to life in general. However, their effect is only short-lived unless they are constantly reinforced.
- **Positive character** – the engaged life. Self-actualization through a process of personal development, such as by

learning, and by honing skills to achieve optimum potential, which is more likely to produce more lasting happiness.
- **Positive institutions** – the meaningful life. The eighteenth-century Scottish philosopher Francis Hutcheson noted that 'Man is never happier than when he is helping others', and this is a very important observation. Serving a 'greater good', whatever that may be, may seem selfless, but there actually seems to be an almost universal facet of human nature that re-sults in it bringing us the greatest long-term happiness, so it can also be considered to be self-satisfying.

Paradoxically, growth and personal life changes are not always perceived as pleasant (Maslow, 1999), because any change is asso-ciated psychologically with loss. Carl Rogers (1961), one of the pi-oneers of humanistic psychology, observed that people who made real progress towards what can be considered 'a good life' would typically not regard themselves as happy or contented, stating

The good life is a process, not a state of being.

Exercise in Goal Setting

Bearing your list of prioritized values from the earlier exercise in this chapter firmly in mind, write down your three most impor-tant long-term goals. Make sure they are SMART – specific; mea-surable; achievable; realistic and timely (although the timescale for life goals may be long). Consider these questions for each goal:

- What will happen if you achieve the goal?
- What will not happen if you achieve the goal?
- What will happen if you do not achieve the goal?
- What will not happen if you do not achieve the goal?

If you are still happy with the three, see if you can begin to for-mulate an action plan of how to reach those goals. Break it down into small, achievable steps.

MISSION

A sense of mission is commonly identified as being an important driver towards excellence, yet to many veterinary professionals the term is off-putting – seen as too evangelical and egocentric. What the term means within this context is that we have a clear idea of the kind of veterinarian we would like to be, the types of things we might do, and the values that we most dearly cherish. A mission is a focusing and articulation of our values and goals, providing a clear blueprint of an idealized plan of our future selves. It is relevant to organizations, as we have already discussed, but it is also important to us as individuals, in terms of fulfilling our potential.

Motivational studies, particularly within the sporting world, have shown that the more clearly we are able to visualize our mission, the more likely we are to be able to achieve it. We can express our mission in words, and doing so is well worthwhile, for if we are unable to articulate it, what hope do we have of passing on to others? But to be effective as a motivating force, we have to not only talk the talk, but walk the walk, and make it clear to others from our actions that we are serious about where we are heading.

MOTIVATION

Motivation is the force that drives us to do the things that we do, and is the organized patterning of our goals, emotions and beliefs (Ford and Nichols, 1991). Thus it depends upon the interrelationship between where we aspire to be, the amount of energy we expend to get there, and our belief in our own ability to succeed.

Motivational drivers can be divided into two main types: intrinsic and extrinsic. Intrinsic motivation reflects the inborn tendency that all humans share to seek out new experiences and challenges, to explore our surroundings, and to stretch our abilities. When we are internally motivated, we do something simply for the sake of it, because we enjoy doing it, so it's pretty easy to persuade ourselves to do them.

Extrinsic motivation can be divided into four subtypes (Ryan and Deci, 2000):

1. External motivation happens when we feel driven by outside forces, to either obtain a reward or avoid a punishment. We do something because we are compelled to do so for external reasons.
2. Introjected motivation is based upon self-control, where we do something because we would feel guilty if we did not.
3. Identified motivation means that we do something because we feel that it is worthwhile and important, even if we don't actively enjoy doing it.
4. Integrated motivation means we do something because we fully subscribe to the values underlying it, which have become part of ourselves.

We see how our consideration of values ties into our motivation, because we are more likely to be happy to carry out a task if we are intrinsically motivated to do so, or if the extrinsic motivation is identified or integrated. If we gain an understanding of what we are doing, and the reasons for doing it, we are therefore likely to be more strongly motivated than if we decide to do it simply to earn a living, avoid punishment, or avoid punishing ourselves with guilt. We need to develop an understanding of how we work best. For example, many of us are more strongly motivated if we work in a group with other, like-minded individuals who are able to offer mutual support and encouragement.

If we choose to do something voluntarily, we are enhancing our intrinsic motivation, and will carry it out more readily. This is why we are likely to be much more strongly motivated in our work if we feel we have a sense of autonomy – a choice of exactly what and how we do things. We shall see in Chapter 6, how effective leadership revolves around developing a workforce whose goals fit in with those of the organization, because that is the only way to get people to perform their jobs effectively in the long term.

In the previous chapter I considered the issue of optimism and its effect upon our performance. Closely related to this issue, is our ability to conceptualize goals, find pathways to reach them, and to persist in our efforts to succeed. Collectively, these abilities combine to produce what Snyder et al. (2002) describe as 'Hope'. Even if the main route to achieving a goal appears blocked, a hopeful person will determinedly find other ways of reaching it. Therefore, motivation is not only about identifying goals and starting out on them, but staying focused upon them. This is a very significant quality that marks out many prominent entrepreneurs and leaders from others, although the personality traits required to visualize goals and start out towards them are not the same as those required to finish the task on hand, and many personality profiles specifically differentiate between 'starters' and 'finishers'. Whatever the scale of the task, it is important that we not only formulate a clear idea of where we are heading, but that we develop an honest self-awareness of our own strengths and weaknesses. This enables us to enlist appropriate support, or develop our own weak areas, in order to succeed.

SUMMARY

In this chapter we have considered the underlying essence of how to achieve happiness within veterinary practice, for it is a fundamental premise of this book that in the long-term success in veterinary practice has to be linked to personal happiness through professional fulfilment. If you are like me and like to conceptualize issues visually, this mind map may help (Figure 3.1).

A mismatch between our underlying values and our life goals, or achieving goals that actually doing not bring us the happiness that we expected, are major causes of work-related stress and professional dissatisfaction.

For long-term satisfaction we need to bring together our values and goals with our current state of reality. Yet the human personality is not quite as simple as that: we must recognize the inherent restlessness of the human mind. Very few of us are able to set realistic goals and then remain serene and appreciative once we have

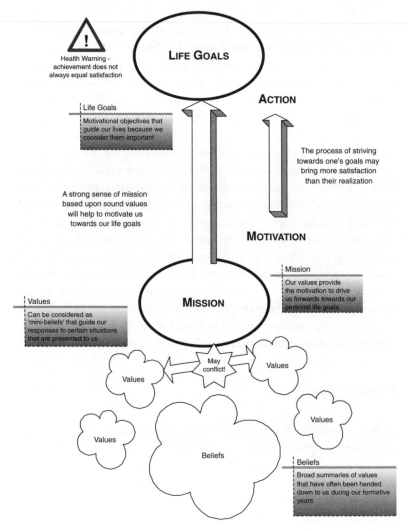

Figure 3.1   Mind map of happiness.

reached them, although that is a skill well worth fostering in its own right. For the rest of us, most often the matching of reality to our own ideal will always remain an objective rather than a reality, either because we set those goals at a level that are never likely to be attainable, or because we re-set our goals as new horizons become visible to us.

If you just want to read one book...

I've put quite a bit of thought into this. I've already mentioned Illona Boniwell's book in the last chapter, which also contains lots of valuable information on beliefs, values and goals.

But the book that I would recommend that is related to this area, indeed, one of the most enlightening I have ever read, is 'The Mind and the Way' by Ajahn Sumedho. He expresses Buddhist philosophy in a manner that is relatively easy for the Western mind to grasp. There is a strong congruence between the practical advice it contains and cognitive therapy, such as a concentration on the 'Here and Now' rather than harping on what has happened or what may be, and it certainly puts goal setting into a broader perspective.

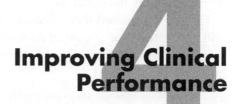

Improving Clinical Performance

This chapter puts into context the application of the clinical knowledge that we have accumulated throughout our training. In a tidy and scientific world all the clinical decisions that we make are based upon a complete set of data, and the diagnostic and treatment options that we decide to follow are founded upon a sound evidence base. Once we complete our undergraduate training, particularly if we go into general practice, we quickly realize that life is just not like that. As we will discuss further in Chapter 7, that is the fundamental difference between undergraduate and postgraduate learning, with the latter seeking to develop competence within the framework of uncertainty that the workplace invariably throws at us.

Having considered these uncertainties, the rest of the chapter will look at the issue of clinical governance, and how the measurement of clinical outcomes can be used to maximize our clinical effectiveness.

EVIDENCE-BASED VETERINARY MEDICINE

The practice of Evidence Based Medicine is a process of lifelong self directed learning in which caring for our own patients creates the need for clinically important information about diagnosis, prognosis, therapy and other clinical and health care issues. (Sackett et al., 1997)[*]

There has been a very significant move in human medicine towards basing clinical decisions upon sound scientific evidence, as driven forwards globally by the Cochrane Collaboration (see www.cochrane.org) which collates systematic reviews of the literature on particular medical interventions. An excellent overview of evidence-based veterinary medicine (EBVM) has been produced by Peter Cockcroft and Mark Holmes (2003).

It involves a five-stage process in which we need to:

1. Convert information needs into answerable questions which may be about:
   a. The patient or problem being addressed
   b. The intervention being considered
   c. A comparison intervention (or control)
   d. The clinical outcome
2. Track down, with maximum efficiency the best evidence with which to answer them (whether from the clinical examination, the diagnostic laboratory, from research evidence or other sources.

---

[*] This extract was published in D.L. Sackett, *Evidence-Based Medicine: How to Practice and Teach EBM*, second edition, © 1997 Elsevier.

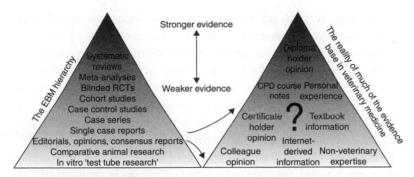

Figure 4.1   Hierarchy of evidence. Reproduced with permission from Cockcroft and Holmes (2003).

3. Critically appraise the evidence for validity (closeness to the truth) and usefulness (clinical applicability).
4. Apply the results of this appraisal to our clinical practice.
5. Evaluate our own performance.

The essence of the process is to recognize that there is a hierarchy of evidence for the treatment that we offer, that can best be visualized as a pyramid with a systematic review of randomized double-blinded trials at the apex (Figure 4.1).

It is vital to recognize that the evidence base for human medicine is only just being established for a wide range of conditions, with the benefit of a great deal of funding. The veterinary scenario is still a long way behind, and in most cases only fragmented evidence exists. That does not mean that we should ignore the principles behind EBVM – we should always make the effort to critically evaluate the quality of the clinical advice that we are given. Once one gets into the habit of doing so, it is amazing how often the perceived wisdom is based upon anecdotal evidence, theoretical hypothesizing of what seems best, or evidence based upon scientifically questionable data. It is hoped that as the veterinary profession wakes up to this fact, there will be an increasing demand upon the research community to provide clinical research that truly meets the needs of practicing veterinarians.

What do we turn to guide our actions when the desired evidence simply does not exist? Isaacs and Fitzgerald take a light-hearted look at the subject in the *British Medical Journal* (1999), identifying several alternative systems, including eminence-based medicine; vehemence-based medicine, and eloquence-based medicine. As is so often the case, many issues taken in jest often rely upon an element of truth to support them, and the decision to support a particular line of treatment is often taken on the basis of advice that is given by someone that we take heed of simply on the basis of their superior experience, forcefulness or sheer persuasiveness. The latter may particularly be the case with the more effective drug company representatives, for how many of us can honestly say that our therapeutic decision making has never been swayed by the silver tongue of a first-class pharmaceutical salesman?

SCIENTIFIC UNCERTAINTY

When considering the evidence behind any clinical decision-making, it is also worth being aware of imperfections that apply to the scientific method. Even apparently well-designed experiments will have intrinsic weaknesses that limit their application. As long ago as 1935, a Polish physician by the name of Ludwik Fleck considered this issue in 'Genesis and Development of a Scientific Fact'. His idea can be illustrated by the problem of over-matching in case–control trials: this experimental design is particularly valuable for investigating causal factors of relatively rare diseases, with the exposure history of affected patients matched with normal controls according to age and gender. In order to make the results meaningful, the cases and the controls need to be matched – comparing the exposure history of a 70-year-old female with a 20-year-old male is not likely to be meaningful, and one could match for a whole variety of factors, such as height, weight, education, occupation, diet and so on.

But the more closely we match the case and control groups, the more likely it is that the two groups will have lived in similar circumstances, and thus been exposed in a similar way to the true causative factors. Since our controls are, by definition, disease-free, it means that they may have some intrinsic resistance to the exposure, compared to the 'normal' subjects who have been unable to resist the risk factor in question. This unwittingly leads to a biased comparison which may lead us to the conclusion that the studied factor is less important, or even not a risk factor at all.

The answer to this conundrum is obvious: we should not match any of the variables that actually cause a part in causing the disease in question, but that means that in order to design the experiment perfectly, we need to know what the causative factors are beforehand, in order to exclude them. A classic Catch 22 situation, where one has to understand to be able to understand, as Fleck explains:

> *All really valuable experiments. . . . are . . . . . uncertain, incomplete, and unique. And when experiments become certain, precise and reproducible at any time, they are no longer necessary for research purposes proper, but function only for demonstration of* ad hoc *determinations. If a research experiment were well defined, it would be altogether unnecessary to perform it. For the experimental arrange ments to be well defined, the outcome must be known in advance; otherwise the procedure cannot be limited and purposeful.*

We also need to be very careful with the way in which the data are interpreted, even if it is formulated as the result of a randomized trial. This was illustrated by Leonard Leibovici (2001) who was able to demonstrate the benefit of what he described as 'retroactive intercessory prayer', where his team prayed for the benefit of patient that had been in their hospital four years previously and showed that they did better than a control group. Rather than being an attempt to demonstrate the power of prayer, it was a tongue-in-cheek exercise to demonstrate the dangers of selecting data to try and prove a point from within a much larger set of data – if we are looking for a statistical significance of 5%, then 1 in 20 studies will show a false-positive correlation. In other words, if we take a large set of data and look for patterns within it, we are very likely to find them, but they are more likely to be random fluctuations than scientific proof of any underlying 'truth'. This bias is further amplified by the fact that results that demonstrate a positive correlation, such as the benefit of a new drug over an old one, rather than a negative one, are far more likely to be presented for publication, particularly if they have been funded by a company that has a vested interest in not publishing unhelpful data.

This does not mean that scientific research is of no value – we all realize that in able to ask *anything* we have to understand *something*.

> *The task of a scientist is not to abandon all prejudices in order to have a perfectly objective attitude to the experimental issues, but rather to be as conscious as possible of his own commitments, to enable him to see the role of his background theories and so avoid wrongly generalizing from them.* (Edmund Husserl)

Even for a laboratory-based experiment, the design of the study, the selection of relevant equipment, the calibration of measuring instruments, and so on, are all based upon assumptions about the nature of the phenomena under study. It may take several false starts with an experiment to realize that there was something wrong with the underlying assumptions that were made, and so the understanding of the phenomena being investigated takes a step forwards and the experimental design can be adjusted accordingly.

UNCERTAINTY IN VETERINARY CARE

To blur the boundaries even further, the quality of the knowledge base behind the interventions that we use is only one potential source of uncertainty. John Saunders (2004), a consultant physician and professor at the Centre for Philosophy, Humanities and Law in Healthcare at the University of Wales, describes four different types of uncertainty, which can be transposed to the veterinary scenario:

1. Uncertainty in communication, or **interpersonal uncertainty**, where issues arise in terms of the passage of information between the owner and the veterinarian, even when they share the same language. This may be due to cultural differences, or due to inhibitions about discussing the real issues underlying the consultation. For example, someone may be thinking about euthanasia because their elderly pet has a combination of problems that make it difficult to live with, but the owner

may not feel able to broach the subject. A further barrier to the effective application of veterinary care may relate to the nature and behaviour of the patient concerned. Many of the animals to which we attend may be uncooperative or even downright aggressive, making clinical examination and treatment difficult.

2. Lack of knowledge, or **uncertainty arising from ignorance**. As discussed above, the veterinarian may not have the knowledge required to diagnose or treat a particular problem. The degree to which a clinician needs to feel certain about the knowledge that they possess will depend upon the gravity of its consequences. For example, if a drug is known to have narrow margins of safety, or if a terminal diagnosis may result in the euthanasia of the patient, the level of certainty will be higher than in many other instances.

3. **Uncertainty in application**. The veterinarian may well know the theory behind the treatment of a case, but may be unsure about the extent to which it applies to the patient in question. I have described the hierarchy of evidence earlier in this chapter, and the better the quality of evidence the more confident the clinician may feel about applying it in particular circumstances. But even where the evidence may be of the highest order, the clinician may be unsure about how well that applies in that particular case. For example, faced with treating a 16-year-old cat with renal disease, there may be randomized double-blinded clinical trials of a particular drug, but it may not have included elderly animals.

4. **Moral uncertainty**. The clinical issues may be clear, but as discussed in the previous chapter, ethical ones may raise problems. A patient may be suffering from an eminently treatable disease, but the owner may be reluctant to carry out any therapy. Is the veterinarian able to square the veterinary commitment to care for the welfare of animals under his or her care, or should the wishes of the owner be picked up upon, and carried out? The degree to which an individual believes in moral certainty, compared to a belief that all morals are relative, will vary greatly depending upon the religious and philosophical stance of the individual.

Living with uncertainty is an inevitable part of clinical practice, and the budding veterinarian needs to make the transition from where everything is seemingly known, but not by him or her, to a world where he or she realizes that the more that is learnt, the more there is to discover. To quote Isaac Newton:

> *I seem to have been only like a boy playing on the seashore and diverting myself in now and then finding a smoother pebble or a prettier shell than ordinary, whilst the great ocean of truth lay all undiscovered before me.*

It is important to bring the decision-making process out of the subconscious and to the forefront of our mind, so that we can reflect upon the various factors, weigh them up realistically, and come to a fully rational decision. These decisions will only rarely be black and white, based upon irrefutable scientific data. More often, they will rely on clinical judgement that can be honed over the years by reflective practice.

An Exercise in EBVM

- Pick a treatment that you use commonly, for example, for congestive heart failure and describe in writing the therapeutic approach that you would use for a particular type of case.
- Do a literature search and investigate any other sources of evidence for the treatment protocol that you use.
- Look really critically at the evidence base and then rate where you would place each piece of it within the hierarchy of evidence as outline above. Don't just take a conclusion as gospel, but look at the quality of the data behind it.
- Evaluate how confident you are about the evidence to back up your treatment protocol.
- Consider if you would like to make any changes in light of the evidence review you have carried out.

CLINICAL GOVERNANCE

Having taken several shots across the bow of the conventional wisdom of scientific method, I now intend to look at a structure that can be used to try and maximize our clinical effectiveness. This rests within the umbrella of clinical governance, which has been defined as

> *A framework through which organizations are accountable for continually improving the quality of their services and safeguarding high standards of care by creating an environment in which excellence in clinical care will flourish.* (Scally and Donaldson, 1998)

Clinical governance is a system for improving the standard of clinical practice. It is about looking at one's own practice, considering how it might be improved, and then implementing the changes and finding out if the changes work. It consists of a series of processes for improving quality and ensuring that professionals are accountable for their practice. It is about creating a 'whole system' cultural change to provide an organization with the means to deliver sustainable, accountable, patient focused, quality-assured clinical care. The following information about veterinary governance and audit has been developed over recent years via my Doctoral studies and the collaborative work of the SPVS Clinical Audit MSc group, to whom I am very grateful for their permission to include their results.

The following seven areas are considered to be the 'pillars' that support clinical governance within an organization:

1. **Risk management** – including compliance with legal requirements – e.g. health and safety legislation, medicines legislation and review of critical events.
2. **Staffing and staff management** – including building of teams committed to improving quality of care and a working environment in which problems can be openly discussed (see Chapter 6).
3. **Patient/client involvement** – including effective communication of the evidence that helps clients to make informed decisions and avoid unrealistic expectations (see Chapter 5).
4. **Education, training and CPD** – the responsibility of professionals to keep up to date and to ensure the training of their staff (see Chapter 7).

5. **Use of information** – including record keeping and evidence-based veterinary medicine.
6. **Clinical effectiveness** – the application of the best available knowledge, derived from research, clinical experience and client preferences to achieve optimum processes and outcomes of care for patients. A process whereby practices can systematically promote (and be seen to be promoting) good clinical care.
7. **Clinical audit** – the systematic review of clinical performance and the refining of clinical practice as a result of measuring performance against agreed criteria. It is a method of measuring clinical effectiveness.

CLINICAL EFFECTIVENESS

Clinical effectiveness is a measure of the extent to which particular interventions achieve the desired outcomes. It has been defined as

> *The application of the best available knowledge, derived from research, clinical experience and patient preferences to achieve optimum processes and outcomes of care for patients.* (Royal College of Nursing, 1996)

Obviously in veterinary practice we need to adapt this definition to take account of 'client' preferences and outcomes for both client and patient. There are three key functions needed to improve the clinical effectiveness of services we provide for our clients and their pets:

- **INFORMING** staff and clients about the available evidence on clinically effective practice.
- **CHANGING** current practice as needed to be more clinically and cost effective.
- **MONITORING** actual practice to see if changes are taking place and services are effective as they can be for all involved.

Methods of Assessing and Improving Clinical Effectiveness

1. **Criterion-based audit cycle** involving defining targets, collecting data to measure current practice against those targets for specific criteria and implementing any changes necessary.
2. **Significant event audit/critical incident review** – peer review of cases which have caused concern or from which there was an unexpected outcome. Discussion and reflection to enable the team to learn from/improve in future. Morbidity and mortality reviews are one example of how significant event auditing can be incorporated into practice.
3. **Peer review** – an assessment of the quality of care provided by a clinical team with a view to improving clinical care, including interesting or unusual cases.
4. **Client survey and focus groups** – methods to obtain users' views about the quality of care they have received.
5. **Benchmarking** – this may be **internal**, that is comparison within a practice or group, **external** – comparison with similar practices or against an externally set '**gold standard**' if such information is available.

CLINICAL AUDIT

Clinical audit sits within the remit of clinical effectiveness, which in turn is part of clinical governance (Figure 4.2).

At its simplest, it is the collecting and recording clinical information with the aim of monitoring the quality of care. Clinical audit is about the quality of care given to patients and it usually involves asking one or more of the following questions:

- Did the patient get better?
- Did we give the best available treatment?
- Did we deliver the treatment in the best possible way?
- Was treatment and care provided in the best possible environment?

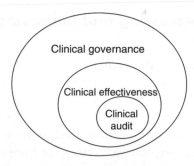

Figure 4.2   How clinical audit fits in.

This can be developed into a systematic review of clinical performance and the refining of clinical practice as the result of measuring performance against agreed guidelines. Therefore clinical audit, when it is done correctly, provides an objective way to review quality within a framework of support and development. It is a powerful tool for creating positive change and a resultant improvement of practice for clients and their animals.

The essence of clinical audit is to develop and improve clinical practice. Although clinical audit might feel like a relatively new concept to the veterinary profession, the belief that clinical staff should be constantly seeking to improve care is as old as the profession itself. Clinical audit takes this concept a step further, and promotes the idea of continuous improvement – ensuring not just good care, but an ongoing process of development, which is known as the 'audit cycle'.

The Audit Cycle

The clinical audit cycle has been defined as (Figure 4.3)

> *A quality improvement process in clinical practice that seeks to establish guidelines for dealing with particular problems, based on documented evidence when it is available, measuring the effectiveness of these guidelines once they have been put into effect, and modifying them as appropriate. It should be an ongoing upward spiral of appraisal and improvement. (Viner, 2006)*

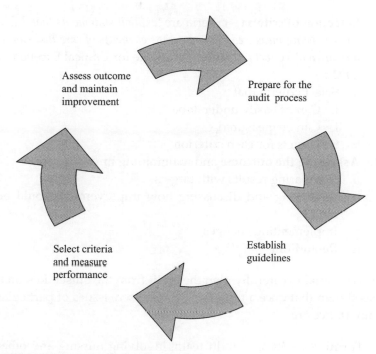

Figure 4.3   The clinical audit cycle.

The 'key' components of the audit cycle are:

1. **Preparation** – this includes:
   a. Selecting an area to audit
   b. Considering your objectives for the audit
   c. Making sure that you are able to record and retrieve information
   d. Involving the team in the process which includes developing a culture in which problems and differences of opinion can be freely discussed
2. **Establishing guidelines** – clinical guidelines are recommendations for the care of patients, based on the best available evidence these should be agreed:
   a. Using the evidence-based literature
   b. Agreeing 'Best Practice' in each practice circumstance

3. **Selection of criteria** – criteria are *'explicit statements that define what is being measured, and represent elements of care that can be measured objectively'* (National Institute for Clinical Excellence, 2002):
   a. Select criteria that
      i. Can be easily understood
      ii. Can be measured
   b. Set targets for each criterion
4. **Assessing the outcome** and maintaining improvement:
   a. Comparing results with targets
   b. Reviewing and discussing how improvements could be made
   c. Implementing changes
   d. Re-auditing

It is essential to carefully plan the audit from the outset. Research has shown that once a topic has been chosen, issues of particular importance are:

- Forming a cohesive audit team, involving nursing and other staff.
- Establishing and communicating clear guidelines informed by the best evidence available.
- Thinking carefully about the type of audit (process or outcome) and establishing clear criteria that can readily be measured.
- Considering the resource implication, particularly demands on time.
- Taking care not to try and run a practice-based research project rather than a clinical audit.

Why Audit?

The primary reason to undertake clinical audit is as a tool to improve our clinical effectiveness, the care that we are able to provide for our patients and the service that we provide to our clients; however, there may be other reasons for undertaking clinical audit such as:

- To find out what we are doing
- To confirm that what we are doing is acceptable and improve job satisfaction
- As a basis for improvement
- To help standardize care throughout the practice
- To increase public confidence in the profession as a whole and in individual practice procedures
- In order to fulfil the requirements any national or local practice standard schemes
- Because if we don't do it, it will be imposed externally on us
- To assist in creating a positive culture within the clinical team
- As a management tool with the potential to increase practice income

Why Not Audit?

Although there are many reasons for and benefits from undertaking audit, there are also barriers:

- Time – it takes time and effort to set up an audit
- Manpower – staff may be taken away from other activities
- Technology – while there is no reason why audit cannot be done with pen and paper it is more frequently carried out using computer data
- Skills – lack of appropriate training
- Money – although there may also be cost benefits as outlined below
- Feeling of loss of control by clinical staff

Research that I carried out within the veterinary profession in the UK (Viner, 2003) identified that they perceived time and financial resources as key barriers to the introduction of clinical audit and reinforced the fact that in order to succeed, sufficient protected time must be made available for the work involved, and this has significant cost implications.

A significant point that arose in my later Doctoral research (Viner, 2006) is that there are also significant benefits that can be gained from the audit process that may help to overcome some of the cost barriers. Using clinical audit as a management tool to enable the whole of the clinical team to improve owner concordance with recommendations for treatment can bring not only major financial benefits to the practice, but also (and importantly from an ethical viewpoint), corresponding welfare benefits to our patients by managing their disease problems more effectively.

What to Audit

Clinical audit is a systematic critical analysis of health care including:

- Procedures used for diagnosis and treatment
- The use of resources
- Outcomes

It is not possible to audit all our clinical activities, but by carefully selecting topics that are particularly important, or liable to improvement, we can improve our performance in those areas. There is also evidence to suggest that by carrying out the process, we can make improvements within the practice culture that may produce benefits in other aspects of our work. To be effective, all aspects of the audit need to be clearly defined, and the temptation to stray into practice-based research needs to be resisted. Team members need to be regularly kept informed of the results of their efforts, and guidelines constantly reinforced, to avoid compliance falling off as initial enthusiasm wanes.

The areas of clinical veterinary practice that are most suited to being audited are:

- Amenable to measurement
- Commonly encountered
- Have room for improvement in performance
- Financially significant to the practice and/or animal owner

Types of Audit

In broad terms audits can be divided into two main groups: **process audits** which look at whether protocols or guideline were followed and **outcome audits** which look at the results that are achieved.

Process audits will often progress naturally from an outcome audit which has been used to establish levels of performance, either internally or externally. If a problem is identified, a process audit will enable the practice to change ways in which the outcomes are being achieved.

When comparing performance between practices, it is generally most practicable to compare outcomes, and not processes, as these are likely to differ significantly, and in most instances there would be little hope of unifying them. However, comparing outcomes allows some degree of benchmarking between practices enabling them to need to carry out internal process audits if they identify a potential problem.

Some conditions may be uncommon, but of particular importance due to the critical nature of the incidents, e.g. unexplained deaths. While these are likely to be infrequent and therefore not suitable for a complete audit within an individual practice, their seriousness should prompt an examination of the circumstances and review of processes, known as a **critical incident review**.

Who Should Carry Out the Audit?

Veterinary and support staff are generally positive to the audit process, providing the whole clinical team are actively involved and feel some degree of ownership of the project.

It is natural that a fall-off in staff enthusiasm and compliance with audit guidelines will tend to occur over time so it is important to be aware of this, and to try and counteract it by regularly feeding back to audit team members the results of their efforts, and reinforcing the need to maintain momentum.

Veterinary nurses and technicians play a leading role in the audit process, providing they receive the appropriate support from management and other members of the clinical team. Care needs to be taken to ensure that any strain caused by the extra workload that the audit process puts upon the team members does not act to negate these benefits. If sufficient protected time is not allowed for those working on the audit team, some resentment may result.

Clinical Audit and Research

Research is concerned with discovering the right thing to do;
audit with ensuring that it is done right. (R. Smith, 1992)

When embarking on clinical audit, it is important to be clear from the start how it differs from practice-based research. Research and audit projects will in fact often look very similar; what differentiates them is the purpose they set out to achieve.

For example:

- A piece of research may examine outcomes of a particular surgical technique in order to arrive at a conclusion as to whether it represents current 'Best Practice'.
- A clinical audit would look at the same technique; however, its purpose would be to see if the recommended surgical method was producing the expected outcomes in your hands in your practice.

The similarities between research and audit are that they both:

- Aim to answer a specific question relating to quality of care
- Can be carried out either retrospectively (historical data) or prospectively (collecting data as care is given)
- Involve careful sampling, questionnaire design and analysis of findings

The differences between clinical audit and research are summarized in Table 4.1. Clinical audit can assist the research process in two ways. Firstly, by highlighting areas where the evidence base is deficient, it can help drive research in a direction that is clinically relevant. Secondly, it is possible for audit data to be collated to provide valuable first opinion data about diseases and their treatment. If audits are carefully designed, they can even feed information into larger research projects that are truly designed to scientifically test hypotheses.

The Problem of Statistical Significance

Statistical significance is important in a scientific experiment which has to be designed with this in mind; a control group has

Table 4.1 Differences between clinical audit and research.

Research	Clinical Audit
Creates new knowledge	Tests care given against knowledge gained
Generally is based on a hypothesis	Measures against criteria
May involve 'experiments' on animals	Should never involve anything beyond clinical management
May need 'ethical' approval	Abides by an ethical framework but doesn't usually require ethical approval
May involve random allocation to different treatment groups, including placebo	Never involves random allocation or the use of placebo
Usually carried out on a large scale over a prolonged period of time	Usually carried out on a relatively small number of cases over a short time span
Rigorous methodology – power calculations for sample sizes, statistical tests etc.	Different methodology from research less need for large sample sizes and statistical significance
Results are generalizable and hence maybe published; aimed at influencing the activities of clinical practice as a whole	Results are only relevant locally, influencing activities of local clinicians and teams; audit process may be of interest to wider and hence audits should still be published

to be formed; the numbers involved have to be large enough to be statistically significant; and ideally there will be some form of blinding to minimize bias. Trying to design an audit along these lines will usually result in failure.

This difference is also reflected in the way in which the data that is generated by an audit should be viewed. If it is viewed as scientific data and the standard tests applied, it is usually very difficult to measure a statistically significant difference between the outcomes before and after the changes were put into place. However, if the data are viewed as performance indicators, and investigated qualitatively in more depth where appropriate, logical actions can be based upon these results. They cannot be 'proven' to be scientifically valid and thus generalizable, but once their effect has been measured with a further review of the audit cycle, they can be used sensibly to guide our actions in an informed manner.

The Role of EBVM in Clinical Audit

As the aim of clinical audit is to improve the clinical effectiveness of our practice it is important that any changes that we make are based on the best available evidence. We will need to refer to the evidence base when planning an audit and drawing up guidelines as well as selecting realistic criteria. It is not possible for us individually to trawl the literature for every condition that is presented, but the audit process provides a structure for this to occur. This search for an evidence base is extremely healthy, and will hopefully encourage the exchange of information between specialists and practitioners to establish mutually agreed guidelines for some of the more common conditions that we encounter. In time, the audit process may help to generate a demand for more clinical research that is specifically geared to the needs of practice.

The lack of a base of comparative data to help set benchmarks, mean that almost nothing currently exists within the veterinary profession. Currently, practices wishing to measure changes in performance brought about by the audit process need to establish a baseline measurement of their own performance, either by studying retrospective data, or running the audit before new guidelines are put into place, and so establish internal targets.

Guidelines and Their Relevance to Veterinary Practice

Clinical guidelines can be defined as systematically developed statements to assist practitioner and client decisions about appropriate health care for patients in specific clinical circumstances. Three key features differentiate them from general clinical advice such as may be given in veterinary texts:

1. They involve an explicit attempt to systematically review the literature on the subject in question for the best available evidence.

2. They represent a consensus in the setting in which they are prepared rather than the opinion of an individual. This may be a 'panel of experts' if they are nationally developed guidelines, or a team of clinical staff if they are guidelines being written or adapted for a local hospital or clinic.
3. The information is presented in a summarized form, often as a series of bullet points, so as to be readily accessible in a clinical situation.

It is further possible to distinguish between 'national' guidelines, which are usually published by a professional body to disseminate the findings of evidence-based medicine as widely and efficiently as possible, and 'local' guidelines, which are applied to reflect the availability of resources and clinician preferences in a particular organization. These local guidelines, which by their nature tend to give much more specific advice, are sometimes referred to as protocols.

Guidelines are becoming common within the medical profession because they can bring a number of benefits:

• They provide recommendations for the treatment and care of people by health professionals.
• They can be used to develop standards to assess the clinical practice of individual health professionals.
• They can be used in the education and training of health professionals.
• They help patients to make informed decisions.
• They improve communication between patient and health professional.

Inevitably such clinical guidelines also take into account the cost effectiveness of health care and in the popular media they have often been associated with cost-cutting and restricting access to potentially useful treatments.

By contrast, very few nationally agreed guidelines exist for the veterinary profession, although the World Small Animal Veterinary Association and the American Animal Hospital Association have drawn up some covering various aspects

of small animal practice, and the British Small Animal Association (www.bsava.com) and the Feline Advisory Bureau
(www.fabvets.org) have produced some for their members in the
UK. Recent research has shown that locally produced guidelines
are increasingly being developed and applied in veterinary practice in the UK (Brown, 2007), partly due to the fact that multi-site
corporately owned practices are becoming more common.

The following questions may help in deciding whether they are
relevant in a particular situation:

- Is there a need to improve our practice, or is there new knowledge we need to incorporate?
- Is the situation encountered often enough in practice to make
  it worthwhile developing guidelines?
- Is there a good evidence base and will it allow us to make recommendations that can be widely generalized?
- Is it an area where we want to carry out clinical audit?

Answering 'yes' to one or more of these questions would suggest
that it may well be appropriate to draw up a clinical guideline.

Tips for carrying out a successful audit:

- Carefully select an appropriate audit team and plan carefully
  from the outset.
- Concentrate on good communications to encourage the prac-
  tice team at all levels to 'buy in' to the concept.
- Be very careful to avoid the tendency to confuse in-practice
  scientific research with audit.
- Avoid trying to achieve too much thus making an audit over-
  complicated.
- Pick an area for audit that occurs commonly and where there
  is thought to be scope for improvement.
- Ensure the audit team are given enough 'protected time' to
  carry out the process.
- Avoid changing the parameters of the audit part way through.
- Ensure you communicate the results of the audit effectively
  and follow through with the findings.

Issues Raise by the Audit Process

While carrying out clinical audit within the practice does not raise the same ethical dilemmas as carrying out experimental research there are some issues that should at least be considered:

- Clinical audit does require an environment in which problems and departures from 'Best Practice' can be freely discussed. In the past veterinary (and human) medicine have shied away from the discussion of problems and the public may still not be ready to accept that performance in health care can be anything other than optimal. However, 'near miss' reporting is now accepted practice in air traffic control where problems are considered as a starting point for improving future performance. Therefore, to improve our clinical effectiveness it is necessary that we as a profession take an honest look at our performance and use problems as an opportunity to learn.
- Within the practice preparation for an audit, including the production of guidelines, should provide the opportunity for discussion of different viewpoints and a review of the evidence; this is within the context that individual clinicians remain responsible for the clinical care of their patients and are required to exercise judgement in their application.
- The aim of clinical audit is to improve clinical effectiveness throughout the practice, but once clinical audit data has been collected it may be that significant differences between individual clinicians will become apparent, and some thought should be given to how the issues raised by this will be handled.
- Once the results of an audit have been collected some consideration will need to be given to failure to achieve targets and the need to improve performance. While there are few ethical problems with trying to improve performance there may be ethical implications for continuing to follow procedures which fail to meet expected targets for 'Best Practice'.
- There will also be issues about how collected data should be used. We have already drawn attention to the problems of the statistical significance of clinical audit data, and extreme care

should be taken in drawing comparisons between practices on the basis of audit. There may be benefits to the profession in organized collation of clinical audit data to enable practices to benchmark their own performance but this will raise issues of confidentiality and the possibility of 'league tables' being created which compare practices.

It has been inevitable that this part of the book has been more instructive than discoursive because clinical audit is a new and relatively technical subject. More information and support on the topic can be found at www.vetaudit.co.uk. We are moving into an era where existing paradigms are increasingly being questioned, and modes of practice are being challenged to justify themselves both in terms of the evidence upon which they are based, and the outcomes which they achieve. The clinical audit cycle does involve a practice in considerable extra work, but there can be very significant benefits in terms of improved owner concordance (Viner, 2006), leading to some compensatory increase in practice turnover, and most importantly of all, very significant benefits in terms of fostering improved team work and a 'no-blame' culture. These are essential for the audit process to function properly, but also bring many other benefits to the way in which the practice performs.

EXERCISE

Consider a clinical process that you regularly do within your practice and ask yourself these questions:

- Are you certain that you are practicing in a way which is clinically effective for the patient? In other words, is your practice based on best available evidence which is applied appropriately in the clinical situation?
- Do you know if any research studies which are relevant to this area of practice? Have you tried to review what is available? Is the research valid?
- Are there any clinical guidelines available which describe good practice based on research findings and/or expert

opinion? If so, are they appropriate for use in your practice or could they be adapted?

- Have you and your colleagues discussed and agreed on what constitutes 'Best Practice'?
- Have you acted to identify areas of your practice that could be improved?
- Have you and your colleagues carried out a clinical audit to confirm that you are following 'Best Practice' on a day-to-day basis?
- Have you then acted to make sustainable improvement?
- Have you shared your experiences in implementing good practice with other clinicians?

Consider which of these actions you feel would be appropriate within your workplace and draw up a work plan to put them into effect. You will also need to consider how you can get other stakeholders in the process.

SUMMARY

This chapter has considered how our veterinary knowledge can best be applied to provide the highest quality of care for our clients and their charges. It started by reviewing evidence-based veterinary medicine, in particular how to carry it out, and how the evidence base for veterinary medicine is relatively deficient compared to its human counterpart.

We went on to take a look at scientific uncertainty and its relevance to veterinary care, and saw that the hard and fast rules that we took as gospel at undergraduate level can very rarely be applied directly to the cases that we see in general practice. This is both frustrating and stimulating because it is what makes practice so challenging.

Clinical governance aims to try and maintain and improve the whole experience that we provide to our clients, and more specifically at how we can optimize our clinical effectiveness to ensure we are using the best processes and achieving the best outcomes of care for the resources that we have available. We can try and apply the best scientific evidence that is available to our work with the application of the clinical audit cycle. It is a relatively new tool that can be used to measure and then improve clinical performance, either in terms of the processes that we use, or the outcomes that we achieve. The underlying concept is simple but it needs careful application to be meaningful. However, if applied carefully it cannot only assure our consumers that we are carrying out our work effectively, but can be a very useful management tool to improve our clinical effectiveness and thus enhance our professional satisfaction.

If you just want to read one book...

You could read my Doctoral thesis (Viner, 2006) if you were a real masochist, but the fast-changing topic lends itself better to a web-based format, and I would strongly recommend you visit www.vetaudit.co.uk to obtain a free guide to clinical effectiveness produced by the clinical audit MSc group as well as a great deal of other information on the topic. If you want a potted review on the application of audit, have a look at the article in *In Practice*, a supplement to the Veterinary Record (Viner, 2009).

Good Communications

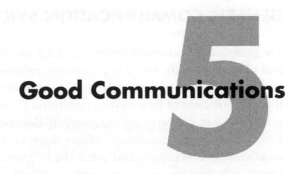

Empathy: the power of understanding and imaginatively enter-ing into another person's feeling. (New Collins Concise English Dictionary)*

Communicating is something that we all do many times every day without giving it much thought, and yet communication breakdowns are the greatest cause of work-related stress, job dis-satisfaction and unhappy clients in any business in general, and veterinary practice in particular. In this chapter we consider the skills that need to be developed to try and ensure good commu-nications occur within our workplace; how to cope when things don't go as planned; and some tips on how to manage the vast amount of information that is thrown at us nowadays.

* This extract was published in *New Collins Concise English Dictionary*.
  © 2007 Harper Collins. Reproduced with permission.

GENERIC COMMUNICATION SKILLS

The purpose of communication is to get a message across clearly and unambiguously, but it is a two-way process that requires effort both on behalf of the sender and the recipient. It's well known that the outcome of face-to-face communications, that are so important within a veterinary consultation, depend more upon non-verbal than verbal messages. When there is a conflict between what someone is saying and what the recipient of that information thinks that the body language is actually saying, the body language is more likely to be believed. Some of us are instinctively better communicators than others, but what is often not appreciated is that it is a skill that can be developed just like any other. Frankel (2006) reviewed the research data on the benefits of improving client communications, and demonstrated a firm link between improved client communications and clinical outcomes in medical practice, as well as a clear benefit of communication skills training. The veterinary research is much more limited, but what there is confirms a similar correlation.

Five Skills to Develop to Improve Communications

- **Self-awareness** of your own communication style. If you are more aware of how others perceive you, you may be able to adapt your style to communicate more effectively. It is worthwhile focusing on what outcome you want to achieve from an interaction, and how best to get there, rather than using it as an opportunity to vent your own emotions, which is usually very counter-productive.
- **Active listening** – as professionals we have a tendency to latch onto the first clues that the people give to us and follow it up with further questions. A lot more information can be gained by giving a person talking to get off their chest everything you want to say. If there is something you want to follow up and are concerned about forgetting what it was, it may help to subtly jot down a word to remind you, but still try and maintain

good eye contact. Increasing the wait time after asking a question, and also after a respondent has finished talking, from an average of one second to three, has been shown (Rowe, 1986) to dramatically increase the interactivity of students within a classroom environment. People want to know more than that you have just heard what they said, they want you to engage with them psychologically, socially and emotionally – no wonder it can seem challenging at times.

- **Giving feedback** so that the person talking feels that you are listening and responding positively – head nodding and 'Aha's' will generally to the trick very nicely, but sometimes a phrase will add emphasis, such as 'I understand how you must feel about that'. Summarizing what someone has told you is an excellent way of confirming that you have been listening and that you have understood it correctly.
- **Non-verbal communication** – if you are in harmony with someone you will tend to mimic their body postures, whereas if you are feeling hostile to what they are saying, you will adopt postures such as folding your arms and leaning away from them. If you become aware of the negative vibes you are sending out, you will automatically correct them if you manage to change your mental approach. Smiling and eye contact are positive gestures, but as already mentioned above, we are all more sensitive to fake messages than we consciously realize, so it largely comes back to emotional intelligence and your approach to issues that challenge you. Similarly, you need to learn to read other people's non-verbal messages so that you can respond to them (Yes, can so often really mean No). Listen with your eyes as well as your ears. Non-verbal cues include:
  - o   Body posture and proximity
  - o   Physical contact
  - o   Body movements
  - o   Facial expressions
  - o   Eye contact
  - o   Vocal clues such as tone, pitch of voice
- **Use of language** – even though we are told that only 20% of communication is verbal in a face-to-face conversation, and 15% in the case of telephone conversations, we sometimes

mis-communicate the words. The use of jargon is easy to fall into, and people we are talking to may not understand the meaning. Alternatively, they may think they understand but actually give words an incorrect meaning – so to many English people 'chronic' means 'really bad' as opposed to its medical meaning of 'long term'.

COMMUNICATIONS WITHIN A VETERINARY CONSULTATION

Veterinarians that have graduated in recent years will have had communication skills taught as part of their curriculum, and there is a welcome move to integrate it further into all aspects of the veterinary course, rather than learning it in isolation. However, many of us currently in practice will have had no formal training at all. Despite more than a quarter of a century in the consulting room doing what I thought was a pretty good job communicating with my clients, I was surprised by how many useful tips I was able to take into the consulting room from reading a medical text about the subject in order to improve my performance.

In the UK, consultation skills are considered such an important factor in the causation of complaints about veterinarians that the Veterinary Defence Society (a cooperative that ensures most UK vets for professional indemnity) has developed a communications training programme with a range of first class material, including a pocket handbook. Their model of the stages in a veterinary consultation builds upon the medical one developed by Silverman and Kurtz known as the NUVACS guide, after the National Unit for the Advancement of Veterinary Communication Skills. This has now been adopted as part of the teaching programme by all the veterinary schools in the UK and Eire, but provides a useful structure for anyone wishing to hone up on their consultation skills.

The NUVACS model lists seven stages, which I briefly describe below, as well as adding just one or two points at each stage that I found particularly valuable:

1. **Preparation**. Familiarization with the pet's history and any relevant details about the client before they enter the consulting room will help to instil confidence, particularly if you were not the last person to examine the patient. Following up on a note made at a previous visit about a non-veterinary matter relating to the client can be an excellent means of rapidly building up a rapport on the next visit.

2. **Opening the consultation**. Niceties such as introducing yourself and shaking hands may seem unnecessary, but can help to make a client feel at ease. Greeting the patient also goes down well with small animals. Beckman and Frankel (1984) published some fascinating research where they observed internal medicine and primary care physicians' consultations and discovered that:

    a. Doctors generally interrupted patients before they had completed their opening statement, after an average of only 18 seconds.

    b. Only 23% of patients were allowed to complete their opening statement, usually because the doctor starts to ask closed questions to hone done upon a particular problem that has been mentioned.

    c. The longer the doctor waited before interrupting the more physical complaints were elicited.

    d. Allowing the patient to finish their opening statement resulted in a decreased number of complications arising later in the consultation.

    e. Most patients who were allowed to complete their opening statement did so within 60 seconds, and all within 150 seconds, even when encouraged to continue.

    f. Previous research had shown that patients did not generally have just one complaint – the mean was between 1.2 and 3.9 depending upon the study. Beckman and Frankel showed that patients did not necessarily mention their most serious problem first.

    At best, this means that information about the patient's concerns are only partly elicited, and serious matters have to be dealt with hurriedly when they arise at the later stages of the consultation. At worst, the patient may leave the consultation without having mentioned some serious medical issues at all. It is to be hoped that since this work was carried out over 20 years ago, before medical communications skills training was commonplace, things have improved now. But communications training has come much later to the veterinary profession, and it seems likely that a lot of this poor communication still goes on. Screening at the end of this stage to check that clients have said everything they want to say is very helpful and emphasizes to the clients that you are really listening to them: 'So what I understand from what you have told me is that Snowy has been out of sorts for the past few days, is eating and drinking normally, but seems to be licking his bottom a lot and is sensitive around his rear end. Is that correct, and is there anything else you would like to tell me about his problems?'

3. **Gathering information**. The vital point here is to actively listen before you start honing down on your clinical suspicions with questions and use all the emotional intelligence that you can muster to try and empathize with your client. Within the context of a medical consultation, it is worthwhile noting the work of Poole and Sanson-Fisher (1979) who demonstrated that medical student's rating for empathy with patients did not improve during the medical course, unless they underwent specific training, in which case significant improvements could be measured. When you do start to ask questions, begin with open ones such as 'What are her bowel movements like?', and then on to closed ones: 'So was there any blood in her stools?' A traditional scientific approach to history taking follows a very systematic organ-based disease model, but with experience this will often be melded with a more patient-centred approach to information gathering, looking at the expression of illness as experienced by the owner and exhibited by the patient (see Chapter 7 for more discussion on clinical decision-making). It is this rich interaction between the bodily function of the patient, its reaction to any disease, and the response of the owner, that make up the totality of the illness, and that is what makes the whole package of signs that we see from the same pathological process so varied. There is no

reason why alternative medicine veterinarians should have a monopoly of looking at their patients and their environment holistically.

4. **Clinical examination**. We're all pretty good at this bit, in fact so slick that the client often does not appreciate what is being done, so it is worth giving a running commentary.

5. **Explaining your findings**. The important part is ensuring that your clients have understood what you told them without sounding patronizing. Putting the onus back on yourself is the smart way to do it: 'Have I explained things clearly enough?', or better still 'Can you run that back to me so that I can see if I have left anything out?'

6. **Planning patient care**. Ensure that you have dealt with the client's initial concerns, even if you have moved away from them. Concentrate on forming a treatment plan that both you and the client are happy to buy into – this process is called concordance, and is more likely to have a successful outcome than simply trying to get a client to comply to what you tell them to do. And don't forget that prognosis is often important to a client, even for what may seem to us to be relatively minor conditions.

7. **Closing the consultation**. This is a chance to run over things one last time, to make arrangements for the next visit, and to make clear what should be done if things don't go as planned – these details should be recorded on the client record as well, in case of dispute. There is often a lot of flexibility as to when cases can be re-booked, so when possible it is best for client continuity to arrange an appointment for a specific day and time when you know you will be available. It is also useful to reinforce your message with specific visual aids such as printed handouts, perhaps with some additional written notes.

Not every consultation is going to fall neatly into this framework, but a structure such as this does act as an aide memoir of what should be included during the course of the normal consultation. The original Calgary–Cambridge medical model developed by Silverman and Kurtz lists 72 skills that need to be covered through the various stages of the consultation. Not every one will be used in every consultation, but they are all important, and medical students are expected to demonstrate competence in them all. This demonstrates how complex the consultation procedure is when it is broken down to its component parts, and how important it is that consultation skills are considered an important set of competences that need to be developed consciously at undergraduate and then postgraduate level.

Doctoral research carried out by Paul Manning (2006) was able to demonstrate a link between and increase in average transaction values and the introduction of consultation skills training to his six-veterinarian practice, as well as a virtual elimination of client complaints. Poor compliance has been indentified (American Animal Hospital Association, 2003) as the major challenge affecting both patient care and practice viability today. Good communications are the major weapon that we possess to combat the problem (the previous chapter demonstrated how clinical audit can be another useful tool in aiding concordance). The AAHA report demonstrated that there was a large gap between what veterinarians were recommending and what clients were actually taking up, and a 10% increase in compliance in a typical 2.2 full-time equivalent veterinarian practice resulted in an additional $132,535 of income and $81,364 of gross profit (at that time). Encouraging clients to follow through effectively with your recommendations for the care of their animals is a win-win situation, with improved standards of care as well as improved profitability.

Dealing with Uncertainty

The old adage that the hardest thing to say is 'I'm sorry' may well be equally true in veterinary practice, but the next hardest thing for a vet to say must be 'I'm not sure what's wrong'. It requires a lot of self-confidence, or sheer desperation, to make this type of admission to our clients, but we often underestimate their appreciation of the processes and difficulties involved in diagnosis. As we shall see in Chapter 7, it is the ability to cope with uncertainty that is one the major factor that distinguishes an expert veterinarian from a novice.

A study that asked both clients and veterinarians from six different companion animal practices in the UK to complete a questionnaire about their feelings about expressions of clinical uncertainty (Mellanby et. al., 2007) came up with some interesting mismatches between the perceptions of clients and their veterinarians. Whereas the vast majority of both clients and veterinarians agreed that it was desirable for the client to know when the diagnosis was uncertain, the veterinarians strongly overestimated the degree to which this expression of uncertainty would result in a reduction in confidence in their ability by the client: 44% of veterinarians thought it would have a negative effect, whereas only 13% of clients thought so, and 34% actually feeling that it would improve their confidence in their vet. The manner in which this uncertainty was expressed was also thought likely to have an effect by both veterinarians and their clients: not surprisingly a blank 'I don't know. . ..' was likely to be poorly received, whereas 'I need to find out more. . ..' was welcomed by both parties. Interestingly, veterinarians very significantly overestimated the loss of client confidence that would result from a statement such as 'I am not sure about this'.

When Things Go Wrong

We have seen above how a lack of clinical decisiveness is rarely a cause for client dissatisfaction if handled well – it's communications that are likely to cause an issue. Work by Tuckett et al. (1985) showed that the most common cause of dissatisfaction with the outcome of a medical consultation was a discordance between the patient's and the doctor's explanatory frameworks – doctors need to explore their patients' viewpoints more fully and incorporate them into their explanations.

There is even more scope for such a difference within the veterinary scenario, where the interests of the patient may not be the same as the interests of the owner. For instance, the owner of a dog with a chronic skin condition may actually not want it to be resolved as they want the euthanized because it is grumpy and sometimes bites them, but is reluctant to say so. On the other hand, a veterinarian may strongly feel that euthanasia is the kindest course of action for an animal with a terminal and potentially painful condition, but the owner may begin with a stance that euthanasia of any animal is morally unacceptable. Resolving the differences may raise ethical issues, but in order to resolve them, communication skills first need to come into play so that they can be clearly identified.

Whatever your role within the veterinary workplace, you are going to have to deal with dissatisfied clients at some stage. Most often complaints arise over communication breakdowns, but sometimes there are genuine issues that can be resolved. The following point may be useful, but every case will be different, and reflection upon such issues in a critical incident diary can be an excellent part of the learning process (see Chapter 8). Some tips you may find helpful:

- Try and avoid the instinctive response to be defensive.
- Think about outcomes – a complaint well handled can result in a highly bonded client, so you can envisage it as an opportunity rather than a threat.
- Try to deal with complaints away from the more public areas of the practice.
- Acknowledge that you understand what a client is complaining about. That is not the same as agreeing with it.
- Apologize for the distress that the client has experienced, for whatever reason. That is not the same as admitting liability.
- Take action that is appropriate to the case, and communicate it clearly to the client. We often think that clients are looking for financial recompense for a problem that has occurred, but very often they simply want to know that the issue has been taken seriously and steps have been taken to prevent it recurring.
- Be aware that a small number of clients are capable of causing you an inordinate amount of grief. There comes a point, particularly with a repeatedly abusive client, where it is best to firmly but politely sever ties with the client.

INFORMATION MANAGEMENT

We live in the age of the information explosion. Since 1960, it is estimated that the number of scientific periodicals has been increasing by about 2% per year. The development of the veterinary specialist clinical divisions has been of particular importance. In the early 1970s, there were around 20 medical journals publishing diagnostic imaging information; by 1978, this number had doubled to around 40 – and today there are 93 such journals listed on Medline. The number of journals in the veterinary field also continues to increase and new journals often focus on one aspect of veterinary interest (Dunn, 2007).

A crucial skill that we need to develop is the filtering of information coming in to us, so that we only spend time looking at data that is likely to be of value. This needs to be accompanied by a recognition that that we increasingly make use of information 'Just in time', rather than information 'Just in case'. The consequence of that is that instead of attending Continuing Professional Development (CPD) courses and attempting to memorize information that we think we might need in future, we just need to be aware of its existence, and where to find it. Information is sought for cases that are presented, and then applied, which uses the time available for CPD far more effectively. The internet now makes vast amounts of information almost instantly accessible and the trend is firmly set for that to continue.

Filtering the Written Word

The first decision to make is whether a particular document is worth reading or not. The art of quickly summing up the value of scientific papers has been neatly summarized by Tom Jefferson, a champion for evidence-based medicine:

If the topic interests you, go to the bottom of the Introduction section. If you cannot find a clearly defined objective, bin the study. Think twice about reading the journal again. If the study has a clear objective go to a results table, add up a column at random and match the results with the total. If they do not match, bin the paper. Remember that if you are adding percentages, the total may be slightly over or under 100%, because of rounding. If you have a little more time read the study backwards starting with the Discussion. If the bits do not fit logically, bin the study. Alternatively match the content of the abstract (the shop window of the paper) with its content. Again bin the study if they do not fit. Crazy? Some wag found errors and discrepancies in a 68% sample of studies.

He goes on it considering some more formal instruments for assessing the validity of research papers, some similar quick and then full instruments for checking out other forms of communication, such as systematic reviews and websites. His site, http://www.attentiallebufale.it/, is well worth a visit. (In Italian slang bufale are red herrings but in real life bufale are female water buffaloes. Their milk is the basic ingredient of the famous mozzarella cheese.)

It's vital to be selective about what we read. We commonly feel an obligation to read every journal that comes in the mail, but all we are likely to end up with is a massive stack of unread journals. Likewise, don't try and read thoroughly every article in every journal that you do decide to read. Think about outcomes. What use is the article likely to be to you? If you think it may have a value, what do you expect to be able to retain in your mind a couple of weeks after you have read it? There are very few articles that require careful reading from beginning to end. Skim the publications, looking at the introduction and the chapter headings in the case of a book, or the summary of a scientific paper.

If your initial survey looks hopeful, you can try speed-reading through the document. Whereas we learn to read letter by letter and then word by word, as adults we naturally learn to scan blocks of text. A poor reader will spend a lot of time reading small blocks of text, and jump backwards and forwards between blocks within a document. It is possible to consciously work upon increasing the number of words that are scanned in each block of text that will lead to faster reading. With training it is possible to reduce the amount of time that is taken to scan each block of text, and reduce the tendency to dart back to previous blocks of text, thus greatly reducing the time it takes to read a document.

Different types of published material will have its content organized in different ways, and if you are familiar with these it becomes easier to pick out the core content:

- News articles try to grab the attention of the reader as quickly as possible, so the important points will usually be at the beginning.
- Opinion articles aim to present one point of view, so the main issues will be outlined in the introduction and then summarized at the end, with the main body of text used to flesh out the content.
- Feature articles are designed to entertain or provide background material for a subject, so the content can usually be found in the main body of text.

Sometimes it is necessary to study a document in detail, and then the emphasis needs to change from ensuring that your attention does not want and you do not start skimming over it. One useful tip, if you own the material or have a printed or photocopied version of it, is to mark the copy as you go, using highlights, underlining and marginal notes to pull the meaning out of the text. Have somewhere where you keep a note of all the information that you think is really important so that you do not have to rummage around indiscriminately to try and retrieve it.

More information on the critical appraisal of scientific articles can be found in Chapter 7.

Communicating by Email

Emails have become one of the key, means of communications within a business context, and have to some extent taken over the use of the telephone, so they are worth a special mention. Utilized effectively they can greatly increase productivity and improve rapid and reliable communication both internally within an organization and externally. However, 'email fatigue' is a major issue due to the sheer volume of emails that many of us receive nowadays. Many of them will be spam, and an effective spam filter is essential, although a balance has to be struck between filtering out as much spam as possible, and not deleting important messages. Getting into the routine of a quick trawl through the junk mail box before deleting them entirely can quickly pick up senders that need to be added to your safe list.

The following tips may be helpful when considering this powerful means of communication:

- Ensure the subject line grabs the attention of the reader and succinctly summarizes the content. This is particularly important if you forward on an email. Emails with blank subject lines are very likely to be deleted without being read.
- Keep each email to one subject. We all tend to deal with emails that can be responded to quickly and easily, and if they become detailed and complicated they are much less likely to elicit a response. It is often better to send several short ones rather than one long one.
- Try and respond promptly to all emails that you consider important enough to warrant a response. You can set programmes such as Outlook to flag up emails from people within your organization, or those that you feel most need a rapid response.
- Emails have a communication style all of their own. Most of the niceties of a letter can be dispensed with, but take care: it is easy to offend by unintentionally making an email sound curt and rude, and once you send one, it forms a permanent written record that can be passed on to others or used in ways that you did not originally intend.

It is worth taking a little time to stop and reflect on how you use emails, and how you can best ensure that they help rather than hinder your workflow. Consider how you organize them within your inboxes to ensure that the important ones get priority and that time is not wasted on those that are not likely to be of any significant value. Their immediacy may distract you from other work that actually requires more urgent attention – some office workers have even got to the stage where they declare 'email-free days', so that other business can be prioritized.

SUMMARY

This chapter has been all about communicating – not just with clients, but with all those with whom we interact in our workplace. Communication has to be a two-way process to be effective, and we have examined certain generic skills that can facilitate that process.

Formal consultation skills training is now well established within the medical profession, and although all veterinary courses now include it, it is still in its relative infancy. The veterinary profession as a whole is not entirely convinced of its importance as a set of competences in its own right, nor is it convinced that they can be learned rather than acquired naturally, but there is plenty of evidence to the contrary. There can be little doubt that effective communication within this area can improve patient care, increase client satisfaction and impact positively upon practice income (Manning, 2006).

There are several different frameworks that have been proposed for veterinary consultations, but the NUVACS one is widely employed and provides a good structure for its various stages. Not every consultation will fall into the same neat pattern, and experienced practitioners will naturally develop their own variations on the theme, but some form of outline does help to ensure that all the components are in place when they are needed.

The importance of listening skills in the consultation process cannot be overstressed, which includes techniques such as supportive comments, positive body language, open questioning, screening, and most importantly of all, letting the client speak, and finish what they have started to say. These techniques have been shown to produce a much fuller picture of the pet, its health, and the expectations and concerns of its owner than a purely systematic approach.

Gathering information effectively is vital, but there comes a stage in the consultation process where it is necessary to impart it, and there is a big gap between what we would like the client to know, what they actually comprehend and then what they translate into action. The American Animal Hospital Association report (2003) identified just how costly poor compliance is, both in terms of finance and patient care. Developing good communication skills has been identified as the major factor governing our clients' concordance with our recommendations. We have also seen evidence of how clients are less concerned about veterinary uncertainty than we think they are, and how effective communications can be used to keep problem cases on the right track, and to deal with them if they should be perceived as going wrong.

The final part of the chapter looked at information management as a whole, for finding, filtering and absorbing what we need from the vast bulk of data that comes our way is one of the major challenges that face all professionals in the modern age. Technology has made it much easier to put our hands on information when we require it, but we need to know what exists, its relative worth, and how to find it. Filtering and speed reading skills can help us to cope with the volume of written material that every professional receives, but there are particular techniques that we can develop to ensure that technologies such as emails become our servants rather than our masters.

The chapter started with a definition of empathy – understanding where someone is coming from and making them aware that they are understood, even if we do not necessarily share their emotions, and I would also like to end there. Despite all the modern technological advances, this basic human skill is crucial to good communications and underpins all good veterinary practice.

If you just want to read one book...

It has to be Silverman and Kurtz. Although written for a medical audience, this highly readable seminal text is packed full of useful information that is directly relevant to veterinary practice. All the advice is founded upon carefully documented evidence rather than supposition.

Silverman, J., Kurtz, S. and Draper, J. (1998). *Skills for Communicating with Patients*. Oxon: Radcliffe Medical Press.

Effective Leadership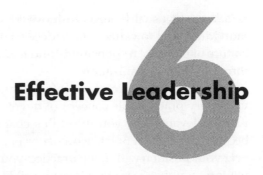

Leadership is about making things possible: management is about making things happen. Lord Bilimoria, founder and CEO of Cobra beer (Courtesy of Lord Bilimoria)

An organization without effective leadership is like a ship without a rudder. It might be thought that by definition a leader leads 'from the front', and is true that many organizations are founded upon the initiatives and policies of a single, strong, individual. However, for an organization to continue to thrive and expand as it matures, it usually needs to move away from the 'cult of the individual' and towards a more decentralized structure, where a culture of personal responsibility and team leadership is devolved throughout the organization.

Within the structure of a professional organization such as a veterinary practice this concept of devolved leadership is particularly relevant, so if you think this chapter is irrelevant to you because you are not practice owner or partner, think again. Whatever your position within the practice, you are almost certain to be working within a team that is responsible for delivering some aspect of client or patient care, and effective team leadership within your own sphere of influence will prove invaluable in assisting you to realize your objectives more effectively.

Within this chapter, I will consider:

1. The meaning of the term 'leadership', and in particular, the difference between leadership and management
2. The relevance of leadership within our workplace
3. The key attributes required for effective leadership and how to develop them
4. The management of change within veterinary practice

WHAT IS LEADERSHIP?

Storey (2004) outlines seven key areas that traditionally define leaders and differentiate them from managers:

1. Leaders need to create new visions. Within a veterinary context, leaders need a clear vision of what they want to achieve, and an understanding of the visions that the other workers within the practice have, so that the two can be fused. This enables workers to find their own personal goals within the overall vision of the practice.
2. Leaders are transformative, i.e. they bring about change. This involves setting a direction based upon a vision that they have developed for the future of the business, and creating an environment within the organization whereby that change can take place. Managers are transactional, which means that they

oversee the mechanics of keeping things running smoothly as they are, or at best, reacting to external forces rather than initiating change.

3. Leaders seek to challenge and change the current systems that are being used, constantly looking for better ways to do things, whereas managers concentrate on ensuring that the current systems run as smoothly as possible.
4. Leaders seek to empower workers to develop their potential, whereas managers are expected to control and monitor them.
5. Leaders should seek to inspire the workforce, whereas managers are more focused upon getting them to do a fair day's work for a fair day's pay.
6. Leaders have a long-term focus, whereas management concentrates more on the short to medium term.
7. Leaders focus on the 'big picture', whereas managers focus more on detail and procedure.

The concept that leadership is different to management has only developed over the past 40 years or so, and in reality the boundaries are not as clear as outlined above. During the course of the 1980s and 1990s there was a great deal of hubris about the development of leadership in the form of charismatic individuals driving organizations forwards and transforming the way in which they carry out their business. To some extent this is still the case, and the airport bookshop shelves are still packed with leadership books, but there has been a move away from this style towards a more devolved model, where leadership is encouraged throughout an organization. In practical terms, this means that workers at all levels take responsibility for their own actions and for their own development, and are encouraged to act with initiative within well-understood parameters.

Storey goes on to explain how transformational leadership, which aspires to significant organizational change through engaged and committed followers, has four components:

• Individualized consideration (the leader is alert to the needs of followers and also takes care to develop them)
• Intellectual stimulation (the leader encourages followers to think in creative ways and propose innovative ideas)

- Inspirational motivation (energizing followers to achieve extraordinary things)
- Idealized influence (offers followers a role model)

Inspirational motivation is particularly central to the concept of transformational leadership. This involves a shift from a supervisory to a strategic direction, and the creation of a learning organization that encourages an experiential learning environment that is inherently capable of evolving to meet the changing demands of the working environment. Inspirational leaders get people excited about a common mission, offering a sense of purpose over and above the pressure of the day-to-day tasks that face everyone in their work. A strong sense of collective mission leaves inspirational leaders free to guide with firmness.

DOES A VETERINARY PRACTICE NEED A LEADER?

What any organization needs is straightforward:

1. A clear idea of exactly what its purpose is
2. A clear mission – a vision of where the business is heading
3. Well recognized and respected values which underpin the way in which it carries out its business with integrity

To achieve that it needs leadership, but not necessarily a leader. The purpose, mission and values can be formulated by a group. In fact, it is important that the mission is formulated with input from the whole workforce, so that they feel able to buy into it. This has to be put into place and communicated continually throughout the organization, but it is not essential for it to be carried out by a single, charismatic leader. If it is not an individual, but say a group of partners, it is absolutely essential that the output is communicated to the rest of the organization as a single clear message. It is this that will create the practice culture and thus the manner in which it operates, as well as its ability to adapt to change, or even drive change forwards.

The distributive model that is now being encouraged is particularly relevant to veterinary practice, because all levels of the workforce are likely to be working in challenging positions that require advanced skills and carry significant responsibility – the junior receptionist that fails to identify an emergency case on the telephone and deal with it appropriately is just as damaging to the practice as a veterinarian that fails to treat it properly.

Caroline Jevring-Bäck in her book *Managing a Veterinary Practice* (2007) considers the evolution of the role of practice principal. In a small practice they act as owner, administrator, manager, leader and clinician, each with their own priorities and requiring their own skill set. As a practice grows, it is becoming increasingly common to hire a practice manager to allow the principal greater freedom to carry on with clinical work, although in many practices the function is more administrative than managerial. As a practice develops further it becomes increasingly important for the principal to fulfil a leadership function, or ensure that it is fulfilled in some other way. This in turn makes it even more important for the practice manager to be delegated full managerial functions to free up the practice leader. Figure 6.1

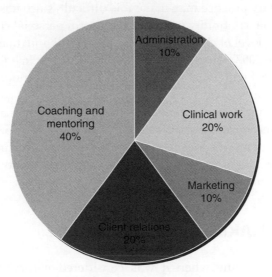

Figure 6.1   Optimum time utilization by a practice leader. After Jevring-Bäck (2007).

illustrates what some might find to be a somewhat surprising suggestion for an optimum division of time for a practice leader, justified on the basis that:

- If more than 10% of time is spent on administration, a trained administrator is required.
- A maximum of 20% for clinical work gives sufficient client contact to keep in touch with developments.
- Not more than 10% on marketing and sales, since the practice leader needs to guide and support practice marketing but the practice manager should carry out the mechanics.
- Twenty per cent of time spent on general client relations includes solving client problems, but more importantly, canvassing clients for their ideas, comments and criticism.
- The most productive use of a leader's time is individual coaching to get the best from staff members – helping staff solve their problems, keep their priorities straight and setting themselves stretching goals and so at least 40% of a leader's time should be spent doing that.

It is interesting to note that performing clinical work is not considered to be the most productive use of time. The personal nature of veterinary practice may make this difficult, since it is challenging to obtain continuity or satisfy long-term personal clients with such a low level of clinical work. On the other hand, many leaders (Leighton, 2007) stress the importance of leaders keeping in first hand contact with what is happening on the 'shop floor', and this has to be the best way for a veterinarian to do so. The concept that a veterinary practice principal working in a function as a leader should concentrate on staff coaching as the highest priority echoes the words of John Storey about the importance of creating a learning organization, but raises issues about the personality traits and skill set required for the task.

WHAT MAKES A GOOD LEADER?

There was a time when it was considered natural that leaders were born, or assumed their position as leader as a right, pertaining to their social status. As social barriers to advancement began to come down, there was still no clear consensus as to what the qualities were that made an individual into a good leader. Characteristics such as statesmanship, integrity, oratory and an ability to unite people were all considered important. Winston Churchill is often quoted as the archetypal 'Great Leader', yet his example is a particularly interesting one, because he was a maverick on the fringes of his political party for much of his career. It was the outbreak of the World War II that enabled him to rise to the fore and demonstrate his not insignificant skills, but his popularity waned again when war was over, and he did not win the first post-war election. He is a good example of how leadership could be claimed to be opportunistic rather than intrinsic – a matter of being the right person, but also at the right time and in the right place.

A report produced by a working group constituted in 2001 (Horne and Steadman-Jones, 2001) by various government departments and DEMOS, the think-tank, was entitled 'Leadership: the challenge for all?' It concluded that the key qualities required by leaders were:

- The ability to inspire (considered absolutely vital)
- Clarity of thinking
- Clarity of communications
- Being able to articulate direction

Pinning down exactly what gives a leadership the ability to inspire its workforce is not easy, but Alan Leighton (2007) finds that one of the key traits that he discovers in his interviews with a series of successful leaders in commerce is a passion for what they do. This translates very well into a veterinary scenario – in whatever practice situation you are working, if you have a passion for practicing good quality veterinary medicine and offering a high level of service to your clients, you will inspire those around you to do likewise. If the key leadership in a practice does not have that passion, it is very unlikely that it will develop from below. Anyone who does have that passion is eventually likely to become de-motivated, and move on to an environment where his or her good work is appreciated. If the leadership do possess a clear vision of what good veterinary practice is about, and a passion to achieve it, but do not communicate that effectively throughout their organization, then it will be largely wasted. This is particularly true in larger organizations, where there is a tendency for the leadership to become isolated from those working at the interface with their customers. It can also easily apply in multi-site veterinary practices, where individual branches become isolated and out of touch with a culture that may have been instilled effectively at a more central site. This demonstrates how communication skills are not only important at the level of our interface with our clients, but also at all levels within a veterinary practice.

Particularly in a profession such as ours, where the workforce are likely to have a strong altruistic element in their desire to work in that sphere, the leadership also requires integrity: an adherence to moral and ethical principles, which returns to the concept of having a sound set of underlying values and sticking to them. If the values upon which a practice are founded are hollow, and just formulated because they sound impressive, this will soon work its way down through the organization. If the leadership expects their workforce to do their job with loyalty and integrity, they have to be prepared to reciprocate.

LEADERSHIP STYLES

There have been many attempts over the years to categorize the different styles of leadership. The reality is that an effective leader will switch between different styles to meet varying challenges, although it is still likely that one style will predominate within the culture of a particular organization. One of the most useful groupings of leadership styles is described by Daniel Goleman in the *Harvard Business Review* (2000), as it is based upon an in-depth analysis of 3871 executives worldwide, carried out by the consulting firm Hay/McBer. As well as defining the styles, it attempted to quantify the effect that each of those styles had upon each of six key factors that affect an organization's performance:

1. Flexibility – lack of unnecessary bureaucracy
2. Responsibility – to the organization as a whole
3. Standards that are set within the organization
4. Rewards – accuracy of feedback and appropriate reward systems
5. Clarity about missions and values
6. Commitment to a common purpose

The coercive style: Dictatorial leadership from the top. Workers are immediately expected to comply with what they have been told to do. This has a markedly depressant effect upon most of the key factors above, especially flexibility and responsibility. People become scared to put their head above the parapet and suggest new ideas, and become resentful of the leadership. There are rare circumstances when this style of leadership is justified, such as in the wake of an emergency situation such as a flood or a fire, or in the short term when a change needs to be imposed upon a failing business. In the long term, the continued use of this style of leadership will have a disastrous effect upon the morale of the workforce.

The affiliative style: This revolves around people, valuing individuals and their emotions more than tasks and goals. An affiliative leader seeks to build such strong emotional bonds with the workforce that they perform well out of loyalty. Communications is usually excellent, because ideas and information are shared freely at all levels, and people are encouraged to work flexibly. The affiliative leader provides ample reward simply by taking an interest in the lives of the workforce, and by offering frequent feedback on progress. The danger is that this approach may allow poor performance to go uncorrected and mediocrity tolerated, so it needs to be used sparingly, in combination with other styles.

The democratic style: This also revolves around people, but in bringing them together to make collaborative decisions. Staff are highly motivated because they have a say in what goals are set and how they should best be achieved. Its overall effect upon the workplace is generally positive, but less than some of the other styles, because decision-making is often weak, and so the message unclear. A significant proportion of the working day may be taken up with meetings to try and reach a consensus.

The pacesetting style: Relies up on the leader setting extremely high standards and exemplifying them – leading by example. The leader is often obsessive about doing things, doing them right, and doing them quickly, and expects everyone else to follow. The vision is often clear in the mind of the leader, but may not be communicated effectively, and initiative is discouraged, as 'the leader knows best' and poor performance is often pounced upon. The style can be effective at bringing about rapid change within an organization, and work well in a highly motivated and competent team that need little guidance, when it will get jobs done efficiently and effectively, but in other situations it can easily lead to micro-management, where the leader tries to ensure that everything is done 'Just so'.

The coaching style: The leader acts more as a counsellor than a traditional boss, listening to the concerns of the workforce and even sharing their own. Coaching leaders help the workforce identify their unique strengths and weaknesses and tie them to their personal and career aspirations. They help them to visualize their own long-term goals and devise a plan to help them work towards it within the organization. They are particularly strong at enhancing the reward and the clarity parameters, and excel at delegating. It is the least often used of the six styles, but works very well if the correct learning culture can be cultivated. Many organizations are coming to appreciate the long-term benefits of this style, and there is a slow move towards it. It is particularly relevant to veterinary practice where ongoing learning is the key to its success, so is developed further below.

The authoritative style: Motivational leadership mobilizing the workforce to follow the leadership towards a strong vision. If driven forwards with enthusiasm and effective communications, it can truly transform the workplace. The research showed that this style of leadership is the most effective at bringing about improvements in all the six parameters. For example, the strong vision enhances clarity so that people understand what is considered important, and since an authoritative leader will be clear about the ends, but allow flexibility in how the workers achieve it, they feel free to be innovative.

Many studies have demonstrated that the more styles a leader is able to utilize, the more effective they are likely to be.

THE LEADER AS COACH

The theme of promoting learning throughout an organization requires that the leaders possess the necessary skills to coach other members of the workforce. These skills are very specific, and very different to the entrepreneurial skills that are needed to establish a new business. For a veterinary practice to succeed as it matures, it is essential that the leadership ensures that they develop those skills.

Coaching requires seven core skills (Dembkowski et al., 2006):

1. Rapport building
2. Active listening (as discussed in the previous chapter)
3. Creative questioning
4. Giving effective feedback
5. Clear goal setting
6. Intuition
7. Presence – the ability to build up a rapport

The coaching process needs to follow several steps, such as:

1. Establish goals of the coaching sessions. Any goals need to be SMART (specific, measurable; achievable; realistic and timely)
2. Appraise the current situation – see below
3. Assess opportunities
4. Plan for desired outcomes including timing and support
5. Review progress

Executive coaching is a rapidly growing industry, and there are many different variations on the basic model outlined above. There are also many different tools used by executive coaches to help their clients clarify their mission – we have already seen the use of wheel of life in Chapter 2 to help visualize work/life not

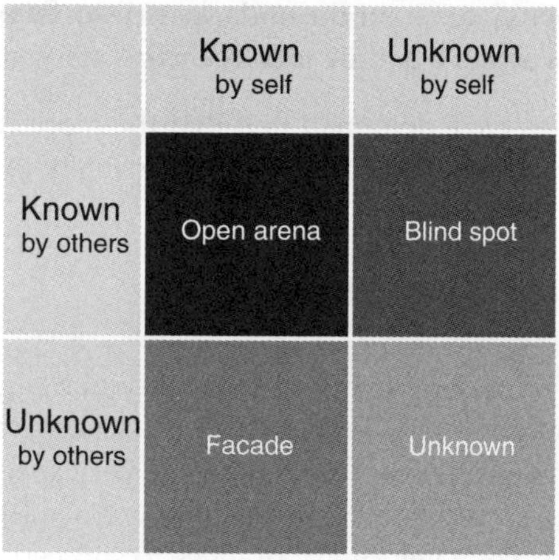

	Known by self	Unknown by self
Known by others	Open arena	Blind spot
Unknown by others	Facade	Unknown

Figure 6.2 Johari window.

live balance issues. Another useful tool to improve self-awareness and develop understanding within a team is the Johari window (Figure 6.2).

The name sounds exotic, but it is actually derived from 'Joe' and 'Harry', the first names of the two psychologists that conceived it in the 1950s, and the concept is similarly simple. The window actually represents information about a person as seen from four perspectives.

The diagram shows the panes of the window to be the same size, but the relative size may alter depending on circumstances. For example, when a team first gets together, the open area is likely to be relatively small, because the members know relatively little about each other, but it will enlarge as they discover more.

- In the open arena, the information is known to everyone involved. Its size can be expanded horizontally into the blind spot, by seeking and actively listening to feedback from other group members. It can also be expanded vertically downwards into the façade by the person's disclosure of information about him or herself to the group, perhaps assisted by sensitive questioning by the group. Top performing organizations tend to have a culture of open, positive communication, so sensitively encouraging the broadening of this area is a fundamental task of effective leadership.

- The blind spot contains information that others in the group know about the individual but of which the individual is not aware. This may be due to ignorance or self-delusion, or it could be because others are deliberately withholding information. Whichever is the case, the aim should be to reduce the size of this area by encouraging individuals to seek feedback, and for other team members to offer it without causing emotional upset. An effective leader will develop a culture that encourages individuals to seek this type of non-judgemental feedback.

- The façade, or hidden self, contains information that the individual conceals from others. It may include sensitivities, fears, hidden agendas, manipulative intentions and secrets – anything that a person knows but does not reveal, for whatever reason. Everyone will always have personal information that will remain hidden, and much if it will not be relevant to the workplace. But some hidden information will be related to work performance and it better brought into the open area through the process of disclosure. Telling others how we feel about issues, and other background information, can lead to better understanding, cooperation, trust, team-working effectiveness and productivity. Organizational culture and working atmosphere have a major influence on group members' preparedness to disclose their hidden selves, which must always be left to the discretion of the individual.

- The information in the unknown area is not known to anyone. Particularly relevant within a practice situation may be unrecognized or underestimated abilities, latent illnesses that are as yet asymptomatic, or repressed, subconscious feelings or past experiences that influence the way in which people react to situations. A healthy organization will encourage a process of self-discovery that will initially bring information in this area into the façade, and in time, into the open area.

Exercise – Using the Johari Window

You can use the Johari window to help improve communications, either on a one-to-one basis, or to help break down barriers within a group. It is vital that it is used with an awareness of personal and cultural sensitivities so that individuals do not feel pressurized to share information that they later regret divulging.

- Give each participant a few copies of the Johari window as per Figure 6.2 – you can easily download them free of charge from the internet if you google the term.
- Also, give each participant a sheet with the following list of adjectives:

> Able, accepting, adaptable, bold, brave, calm, caring, cheerful, clever, complex, confident, dependable, dignified, energetic, extroverted, friendly, giving, happy, helpful, idealistic, independent, ingenious, intelligent, introverted, kind, knowledgeable, logical, loving, mature, modest, nervous, observant, organized, patient, powerful, proud, quiet, reflective, relaxed, religious, responsive, searching, self-assertive, self-conscious, sensible, sentimental, shy, silly, spontaneous, sympathetic, tense, trustworthy, warm, wise and witty.

- The subject and each of his or her peers choose about six of the adjectives that best apply to the subject, and place them wherever they feel is appropriate on their copy of a Johari window.
- Each participant transposes his or her selection onto a copy of the window that everyone can see. The placing of a particular adjective depends upon who uses it:
  - o Those used by the subject and peers go into the open arena
  - o Those used by the subject alone go into the façade
  - o Those used by the peers only go into the blind spot
  - o Those unselected by anyone potentially go into the unknown area
- Use the descriptions for each quadrant as outlined previously to discuss the adjectives that have been used and to try and sensitively enlarge the open arena by the sharing of information.

DEVOLVING COACHING SKILLS

Within a highly successful practice coaching skills will not just exist at the top, but will be devolved down through the clinical teams. The leadership skills outlined above can be applied to a veterinarian working as an assistant in his or her own particular environment, or indeed, any other member of the practice. The larger an organization gets, the more important it becomes to develop leadership skills throughout the strata of its hierarchy. Thus there is a move, particularly in professional businesses, for them to become less vertically hierarchical and more horizontally team-based.

Sound leadership in a modern practice should be all about empowering the workforce to develop their full potential, and an employee that wishes to thrive within such a forward-thinking organization should be looking to see how they can play a role in using their leadership skills to enhance the working of their clinical team. The inculcation of such a culture is not simple or short term, but it is vital if a practice of any size is to optimize the development of its workforce. We must never forget that we are service industry, so the product that we offer to our consumers is the output of the people that we employ. They are by far our most precious asset and success in veterinary practice revolves around developing the competency of ourselves and those around us. In that way we can best meet the changing external forces that challenge us, and turn threats into opportunities.

You will note that the skills that are required to bring about such changes are not primarily technical or purely intellectual, but related to the ability of the leader to tune into the emotional needs of his or her co-workers. This theme is eloquently developed by Daniel Goleman in his book *The New Leaders* (2007), where he reports on research demonstrating that emotional intelligence accounts for over 80% of the competencies that distinguish outstanding from average leaders. He argues that this occurs when a leader creates *resonance* – a reservoir of positivity that frees the best in people. He sees the job of the leader primarily as a group's emotional guide – the individual with the maximum power to sway everyone's emotions. The more emotionally demanding the work, the more empathetic and supportive the leader needs to be – and nobody can claim that veterinary work is not emotionally demanding! We have discussed the topic of emotional intelligence and how to develop it in Chapter 2, but the key is that it is not just *what* we do, but *how* we do it, that influences the effect that our actions have upon a group that is looking to us for leadership. There is no single path to effective leadership: superb leaders can possess very different management styles. Highly effective leaders typically show a particularly high strength in about six of the areas of EI competence outlined in Figure 2.2, although they usually include at least one competence from one of the four fundamental groupings (McClelland, 1998).

Exercise

Reflect upon one core area of your work and consider your role as part of the clinical team. List the key activities involved in effectively completing those tasks, and your role in each. Consider what steps you need to take to try and optimize the performance of your team, and to what extent they involve management and to what extent leadership.

CHANGE MANAGEMENT

However much we are drawn to the familiar, one thing is for sure – the environment within which we work will change, and with that change will come challenges. Some of those challenges can be foreseen, and others will take us by surprise. There are three ways to respond to change:

1. Ignore it: This is very tempting, as it is the line of least resistance, and we are always prone to believing that things can continue as they always did before. But those that cannot adapt to change are destined to become as extinct as the dinosaurs.
2. Adapt to it: Flexibility and an ability to change in response to external changes are vital for survival.
3. Lead change: Only few individuals or organizations will fall into this exceptional category, but doing so enables one to

become a market leader, a trendsetter, and potentially extremely successful.

In *Managing Change in Organizations* (1999), Carnall explains that effective change requires three things from those involved:

1. Awareness – an understanding of the vision and strategy
2. Capability – the skills and resources required
3. Inclusion – choosing to buy in because they believe in the benefits

This is far more likely to happen if this is driven horizontally, at the point of service, rather than vertically, from management above.

Carnall continues by outlining the blocks to change, which in outline can be:

- **Perceptual** – difficulty in identifying the problem, information overload
- **Emotional** – fear of risk, of lack of black and white, pre-judging outcomes
- **Cultural** – lack of intuition, conflict with traditional values
- **Environmental** – lack of support, defensiveness, overbearing managers
- **Cognitive** – jargon, inflexibility, lack of information

In *The Dance of Change* (1999), Peter Senge defines 'profound changes' in this context as organizational changes that combine inner shifts with people's values, aspirations and behaviours with outer shifts in processes, strategies, practices and systems. He proposes that it is not possible to effectively make profound outer changes without equally profound inner ones.

He continues to explain that training implies control but learning is *'enhancing capacity through experience gained following a track or discipline. Learning always occurs over time and in real life contexts, not in classrooms or training sessions'.*

The practice of organisational learning involves developing tangible activities: new governing ideas, innovations in infrastructure and new management methods and tools for changing the way people conduct their work. Given the opportunity to take part in these new activities, people will develop an enduring capability for change. The process will pay back the organisation with far greater levels of diversity, commitment, innovation and talent.

The importance of fostering an environment where work-based learning becomes ingrained within the organizational culture should not be underestimated.

Senge describes three steps to producing profound change within an organization:

1. **Team building** – which requires the recruitment of pragmatists that have a practical approach to the required process.
2. **Spread** – within the organization, built on demonstrable results that benefit both the individuals concerned and the business as a whole.
3. **Developing learning capabilities** – maintaining the maxim 'This is the way I see it', rather than 'This is the way it is', to encourage consensus rather than dogma.

The most important factor governing the success of any business is its ability to develop into a learning organization. This was defined by Peter Senge in 1990 as:

> *...organizations where people continually expand their capacity to create the results they truly desire, where new and expansive patterns of thinking are nurtured, where collective aspiration is set free, and where people are continually learning to see the whole together.*

The most striking characteristic of our modern society is the speed at which change occurs, and it is only by creating an environment where experiential learning is cherished at all levels, that a business organization of any size can develop the ability to adapt to such changes, and turn threats into opportunities.

Some Tips for Effectively Bringing About Change Within Your Practice

- Be clear about the need for change, as part of an overall practice mission, rather than just change for change's sake.

- Develop a 'no blame' culture where everyone is receptive to constructive criticism as to how to do a job better, without feeling threatened.
- Promote team working, where everyone involved in a process understands their importance and takes responsibility for their actions.
- Encourage all the team members to have an input into what changes occur and how. Veterinary practices are not democracies, but if workers at all levels feel their input is valued, they will be far more likely to buy into any change process.
- Structure practice meetings carefully to impart information and to promote feedback. An honest and open approach to the issues involved is far more likely to receive a cooperative response.
- Acknowledge the extra training and time commitment that might be required in order to bring the required change about, and ensure that the necessary resources are made available.
- Whenever possible, set a specific and realistic timescale for changes, and report back the outcomes. Measuring the change, such as by using the clinical audit process described in Chapter 4, can be a very strong motivator.

Exercise in Change Management

- From the previous leadership exercise you should be able to identify some issues within your working environment that require you, as a leader to initiate change.
- Draw up some SMART objectives that are uncomplicated and easy to measure.
- Consider the style of leadership that is most suited to your own personality and the particular circumstances, and then using the tips listed above, devise a strategy for bringing about the desired changes.
- Return to your original notes a couple of months after you have started the change process, and try to objectively measure your progress. If you have failed to make satisfactory progress in all areas, review your strategy and modify it accordingly.

SUMMARY

The situation of leadership within veterinary practice is somewhat different to many other organizations, although this is changing as we see a move of at least part of the sector towards a corporate model in most areas of the Western world. Historically, what has happened is that either veterinarians with drive and entrepreneurial flair have opened up their own practices, which have then evolved and often grown, or junior veterinarians have bought into partnerships, and eventually assumed leadership on the basis of seniority. Sometimes this has worked well, but often it has been a major barrier to the optimization of good veterinary practice, primarily because the skills that have brought veterinarians to the fore as entrepreneurs and/or good clinicians are very different to the skills that are required to provide effective leadership in the modern world. In an environment where the demand for veterinary services is strong, practices can afford to have ineffective leadership and still survive, but the challenges facing veterinary practice in most areas are getting stronger due to increased competition, expectations from the consumers of our services and expectations of the workforce as to what they want to achieve from their work and how far they are prepared to allow it to impinge on the rest of their lives.

We have gained an understanding of how leadership is different from management. Although the same person may sometimes share tasks, the skill set required for the two is very different, and in an organization of any size the roles need to be separated. Having said that, there is now a move away from charismatic leadership at the helm of an organization, towards a more devolved form of leadership, so people who have managerial functions within the organizations are also encouraged to develop leadership skills within the team in which they work. These leaders need the vision to see where they are heading, and the ability to motivate, guide, inspire and persuade their co-workers to strive towards it, and in order to do that they need to be in tune with their emotional needs. Coaching others within the workplace to help them achieve these goals is a key part of the leadership role. Every member needs to be able to work responsibly and autonomously, providing that the leadership in ultimate control has created a culture where everyone fully understands the mission of the organization, its values, the nature of what it is offering and their role in assisting that process.

That last sentence encapsulates everything that is likely to make a modern organization successful, and if it was that simple, everyone would be doing it. Yet when you look around yourself in the role of a consumer, you will see how often that is not the case, and you will see workers who are poorly motivated and poorly informed, and therefore offering a poor level of service.

The key to putting this into place is to create a learning organization, and I make no excuses for repeating the words of Peter Senge, for they are absolutely vital to building a successful practice, where our co-workers are the main resource. He defines them as:

> ...*organizations where people continually expand their capacity to create the results they truly desire, where new and expansive patterns of thinking are nurtured, where collective aspiration is set free, and where people are continually learning to see the whole together.*

Not every employee will want to fit into that mould, but a surprising number will not only rise to the challenge, but grow wings and fly. Refining our emotional intelligence will help to bring us in tune with our colleagues and help us to find the most effective path to draw them towards a shared vision. They will only work effectively if it fulfils their personal goals, rather than those imposed upon them, so an important part of leadership is establishing common goals and driving them forwards. Those that have no interest in their self-development will play a minor role within a learning organization, and most will leave to find a culture that suits them better, but in the long run that will be healthy for the practice rather than detrimental.

So, we see that a key skill that a leader needs to develop, at whatever level he or she is within a veterinary practice, is the ability to coach other members of the practice team, and to continually learn new knowledge and how to apply it in practice themselves. Which leads us neatly on to the next chapter.

If you just want to read one book...

There is much written about the subject of leadership, and much of it is rubbish. John Storey's book is a scholarly publication that can be quite hard going at times, but it is worth persevering as it really does shed some authoritative light on the subject.

Storey, J. (2004). *Leadership in Organizations: Current Issues and Key Trends*. London: Routledge.

Postgraduate Learning

7

The dogmas of the past are inadequate to the stormy present... we must think anew and act anew. (Abraham Lincoln)

What has emerged strongly so far is that the key to good veterinary practice is learning. It is only by continually learning that we can develop as practitioners. Once we think that we know all we need to know, or care no more about everything unlearned, it is time to retire.

In Chapter 4, we considered how the nature of veterinary factual knowledge is often less certain than we would like it to be, with many of our 'truths' actually based upon assumptions. This chapter starts out with a consideration of the nature of different types of knowledge and how best to develop them within our workplace. In particular we will consider the difference between experience and experiential learning, as the two are often confused. We will look at the influence of our undergraduate training on our learning, the transition to postgraduate learning in practice, and how to translate that into effective continuing professional development (CPD).

The synthesis of a whole raft of knowledge into the act of clinical decision-making is something that those of us in practice do many times every day without sparing much thought to the process itself, yet we shall see that the cognitive processes that underlying are surprisingly complex, and only partly understood. Professional competence surely has to be an integral part of what good veterinary practice is all about, so we examine the meaning of professional competence and expertise, in order to better understand how to develop it, as well as the generation of new knowledge from practice.

THE NATURE OF KNOWLEDGE

For our purposes, knowledge can be defined as 'information that works'. There are three types of knowledge that are important to our professional work:

- Propositional knowledge that underpins professional action – 'knowing that'
- Technical skills – 'knowing how'
- Tacit knowledge – what we know intuitively but cannot express

Learning and using professional knowledge are part of the same process that can be hard to artificially separate – practitioners will visualize the application of a new technique when it is described to them. One very rarely learns how to carry out a new procedure without applying an understanding of the fundamental principles involved, but it is important to appreciate that learned knowledge becomes transformed when it is applied. This is because every case that we deal with is different to the last, not only due to individual case variation, but also due to the varying contexts within which it occurs.

There are two fundamentally opposed philosophical stances about the nature of knowledge. The first can be described as the 'brick wall' model, where the knowledge base is considered to be clear-cut. It is assumed that if the teacher presents the students with all the key building blocks of information, and if they are reasonably accurately absorbed by the students, then that information can be recalled when needed to deal with real life situations. We know how even the most scientifically 'black and white' veterinary knowledge has an irritating tendency to become gray once we try to apply it in practice, and that for a great deal of veterinary practice a really sound evidence base for our practice simply does not exist. Yet it is assumed that the teacher is familiar with all these 'bricks' of information, and knows how they fit into the correct pattern to construct a functional model. If incorrect 'bricks' of information are found, such as during assessment, they can be replaced with correct ones. Learning equates to instruction.

It is now widely accepted by educationalists that this traditional model of learning has very limited application within an environment such as postgraduate professional practice. It fails to recognize the fluid nature of knowledge itself and the way in which the vast majority of our learning in practice takes place without active teaching being involved. Teaching is not necessarily the most effective route to learning.

The constructivist model of learning is now generally accepted as being far more valid within the context of a working environment. It focuses on our activities as learners making sense of our world and meeting the demands of the challenges that it presents to us. Our knowledge base is visualized as a vast and flexible network, so that accumulation of 'bricks' of knowledge is just seen as part of the issue. The pattern of information is dynamic, sometimes changing without the addition of new material from outside the learner. Even more importantly, the key to successful learning is seen to be the ability to make sense of this cognitive structure.

This attribution of meaning to information is a personal construct, and experience of their application is essential to developing them to enable us to function efficiently without going back to basic principles every time we are faced with a problem to solve.

LEARNING FROM EXPERIENCE

A physician may have experience but no understanding; a theoretician may have understanding but no experience, and a true expert will have a blend of both knowledge and experience. (Aristotle, 1990; Metaphysics I, 981a–981b)

Perhaps intellectualizing our thought processes may seem to be over-complicating a skill that we have developed through our careers, and has come to a point where it meets our needs. Could it be like getting someone to consciously think about all the unconscious thought processes and muscular movements of the various parts of our anatomy that enable us to stand and walk, to the point where they discover that the task is so complex that they just collapse onto the floor? Thankfully, we are able to learn from experience, enabling us to figure out how to perform tasks without needing to intellectualize the process, just like a small child first pulling up into an upright position and taking those first wobbly steps. Although learning in this way is an intrinsic skill that occurs subconsciously, by increasing our self-awareness of the process we can take it to a higher level. Taking the analogy of walking further, many of us develop back pain later in life due to poor posture, and by consciously improving our self-awareness of our body with disciplines such as yoga or the Alexander technique, we can improve even such basic skills such as standing upright.

It is misleading to equate experience with learning. Experience can lead us to learn a hundred new things, or the same thing a hundred times over, depending upon how we harness it. We romantically associate wisdom with advancing years, and there are undoubtedly very elderly people who are extremely wise. But it is very easy to become increasingly narrow-minded and out of touch with current thinking, and experience can easily serve to reinforce bad habits instead of developing more effective ones if it is not combined with internal and external review.

Once we graduate there is a natural tendency to heave a sigh of relief that our education is over, and then quickly realize that it has only just begun. We assume that learning and developing skills will follow naturally from experience, and that the formalized learning that we need to do involves primarily refreshing and updating our technical knowledge. Whilst maintaining an appropriate knowledge base for the work that we do is essential, by learning how to learn and how to apply that learning to our work we can become much more effective professionals.

The process of applying our internal experience in terms of relevant prior knowledge and past experience and matching it with our current external experiences is fundamental to the concept of experiential learning and reflective practice. The skills involved in the process can be developed, but the learning itself is personal and cannot be taught.

Sometimes new learning may not only have an effect upon our existing state of knowledge, but may also challenge our underlying values and beliefs. For example, the perceived wisdom around the time that I qualified was that cats did not feel pain to the same extent as other species, such as the dog, and it was hypothesized that this was due to the production of endogenous endorphins that have a potent analgesic effect. This was based upon the observation of feline behaviour post-trauma, when they did not demonstrate vocalization and other overt signs of pain in the same way as their canine counterparts, and also because of their different response to canine dose rates of opiate analgesics. More recently, I have had to re-evaluate this belief when new data demonstrated that cats certainly do show physiological and behavioural signs caused by pain, but their overt manifestation is different to that of dogs. Like many other small animal practitioners, I found that I needed to change my perioperative protocols for cats, their post-trauma management, and the advice that I passed on to owners. The acceptance of new knowledge that is at odds with our current thinking is called 'cognitive dissonance' and can be very disturbing if it causes us to have to re-evaluate our personal truths.

This transformational nature of new or internally reinterpreted knowledge is the key to professional learning – it needs to be translated into a change in the way in which we carry out our work, or the way in which we look at issues. Our learning is neither fully rational nor completely haphazard, but is mediated by a mixture of conscious and unconscious forces that will serve us better if we seek to understand how they work. 'Learning to learn' is, ironically, not something that we are generally taught during our formal education, yet it is one of the most important skills that we can develop.

This approach to learning does not denigrate the value of memorizing certain core technical information, but this memorization is likely to be far more effective if it is carried out as part of the process of trying to understand the key meaning underneath the information rather than just as factual data.

LEARNING EXERCISE

I have used changes in our understanding of analgesia in cats as an example of how new knowledge may be assimilated and then applied to our work. Try and think of three more examples relevant to your own work, where new knowledge has caused you to rethink the way in which you handle cases. Think about the following issues:

- Where did you discover the new information? Was it from a single source in a 'Eureka moment', or was did it build up gradually from a variety of different sources?
- How questioning were you of the quality of the new information? What convinced you that there was sufficient evidence to rethink your existing practice?
- What was your attitude to receiving new information that challenged your existing practice, and how did you incorporate it into your daily work?
- How easy was it to change your work routines, and how successful do you think you have been in changing the way in which you do things in your workplace?

The Influence of Undergraduate Training

Undergraduate veterinary education is certainly changing, although some of the changes are negative ones relating to the demands of financial pressures rather than that of producing a graduate best fitted to meet that demands that she, or just occasionally, he, will be likely to face in the Big Wide World. Compared to many of the medical courses, the veterinary degrees are still largely geared to imparting and examining the acquisition of knowledge rather than fostering learning, although there has been a general move in that latter direction.

It could be convincingly argued that those of us who have been qualified for any length of time were victims of our undergraduate courses. They were not primarily directed at encouraging us to think clearly, so they could not be correctly defined as an education. On the contrary, the pressure that has traditionally been put upon veterinary students to accumulate and then regurgitate vast quantities of facts upon demand are likely to have had a suppressive effect upon any natural instincts of curiosity and enquiry that we may have brought with us into the course.

More recently, an over-reliance on the Multiple Choice Question format for assessment may have brought about an increased reliability, not to mention a decrease in cost, but has seriously distorted learning by placing an undue emphasis on the retention of factual knowledge. Although the emphasis on many of the courses is moving towards problem-based learning (PBL), it has to be recognized that for the overworked and highly pressurized veterinary student, assessment is by far the strongest motivation for what is taken from the course. For PBL to be the driver for learning and for self-directed learning skills to be developed, the outcomes of PBL projects have to form a significant part of the assessment process. Veterinary schools tend to dislike this, because the objective assessment of portfolio-based work requires specific training and skills, and is relatively labour-intensive. It also requires very careful planning of the course to ensure that the learning objectives are clearly spelled out.

A balanced education needs to impart three things:

1. The acquisition of propositional knowledge. This is relatively easy to teach, and straightforward to assess, so the veterinary schools have historically done it very well.
2. The development of technical skills. Traditionally this has been patchily achieved, particularly by extramural studies, and very poorly assessed, because it is difficult to do so. Significant strides have been taken in the assessment of such skills, but pressures upon placements due to the increasing number of veterinary graduates, and the decreasing number of certain types of practice in some areas (particularly agricultural practice), have meant that 'hands-on' experience may become an increasingly precious commodity, and artificial alternatives within practical skills laboratories are having to be developed. But these skills amount to more than just the clinical skills that professionals require. They also include cognitive skills such as those we need to find and process information and pass information on to others.
3. The development of attitudes. This is the hardest area of all to impart and to assess, and so it has been largely put to one side. Yet arguably, turning out graduates with suitable attitudes and values to equip them for the challenges that they are likely to face is one of the most valuable gifts that a balanced education can impart.

These shortcomings in veterinary education not only fail to prepare our graduates adequately for practice, but also leave some attitudinal biases which interfere with our postgraduate professional and personal development. These include:

*   A preference for passive learning, where we are told what someone believes we need to know.
*   A preference for learning new facts rather than acquiring new skills.
*   An assumption that one learns best from clinical specialists rather than practitioner colleagues.
*   A narrowness of vision that discourages us from considering learning from other disciplines such as psychology,

philosophy, sociology or economics, which may not be directly related to our clinical practice but nevertheless impinge greatly upon our day-to-day work.

We are more likely to achieve our goal of improving professional performance if we recognize postgraduate education as a form of quest, where as mature professionals we possess the motivation and the means to identify our own learning objectives and strive to meet them.

Some Concepts to Aid Postgraduate Learning

1. Knowledge that 'really' matters – the wisdom that endures and is transferable to every situation – is already latent within us from the outset; specific details can be acquired externally as needed.
2. The task of education in providing an environment in which our capacity for self-transformation can be realized, and self-selected goals accomplished.
3. The role of teacher as that of facilitator, not provider.
4. As a learner, our natural state is curiosity; we sense, subliminally at first, our own needs, and our learning should be focused towards meeting them.
5. The need to guard against the tendency to look for short cuts in the form of instruction from 'experts'.
6. The need to appreciate that there are many different styles of learning, and develop an awareness of which suits us best. This is not necessarily the easiest or the one to which we are most accustomed, as we must carefully consider which are best suited to meet our desired learning outcomes.
7. Professional learning is all about changing the way that we do things. We may attend an enjoyable and comprehensive weekend course on a subject dear to our hearts, but if we return to our workplace and carry on doing everything just as we had been doing it before we attended the course, nothing of professional value has been achieved.

WHAT ARE THE CHARACTERISTICS OF A COMPETENT PROFESSIONAL?

The concept of **competence**, and competencies that involve the ability to carry out specific tasks, or behaviour patterns, can be confusing. This is because the word competent in common parlance can be complimentary, as in 'He's a competent surgeon', or it can be taken to mean that someone has reached a basic level of skill, such as in the Day One Competences that are expected of new graduates. Used in this way it can have mildly derogatory implications, meaning adequate but less than excellent – a client might be satisfied to have someone competent in administering injections to inject their cat, but they might desire something better than bare competence of a surgeon who was going to carry out a complex operation on their pet. It also suggests 'all-or-nothingness', for surely if someone is not competent, they are incompetent, yet in reality there is usually not a clear threshold between the two states.

There is also a difference between competence and **performance** – competence is an assessment of someone's ability to carry out a particular task under optimal, or at least normal, conditions. Performance is how that person manages in a real life situation, so someone may have proven themselves competent to carry out a task but fail to demonstrate that competence when performing the task under particular circumstances. Performance is best assessed by the measurement of outcomes in the workplace, or if impracticable, by simulations that are as realistic as possible.

Work by Dreyfus and Dreyfus (1986) looked at the concept of the development of skills, and rather than accepting the binary concept of competence, defined a model with five levels of expertise. Considering them helps to give us some understanding of how our professional abilities might develop:

Level 1 Novice
- Rigid adherence to taught rules or plans
- Little situational perception
- No discretionary judgement

Level 2 Advanced Beginner
- Guidelines for actions based on attributes or aspects (global characteristics of situations recognizable only after some prior experience)
- Situational perception still limited
- All attributes and aspects are treated separately and given equal importance

Level 3 Competent
- Copes with 'crowdedness'
- Sees actions at least partially in terms of longer-term goals
- Conscious, deliberate planning
- Standardized and routine procedures

Level 4 Proficient
- See situations holistically rather in terms of aspects
- Sees what is most important in a situation
- Perceives deviations from the normal pattern
- Decision-making less laboured
- Uses maxims for guidance, whose meaning varies according to the situation

Level 5 Expert
- No longer relies on rules, guidelines or maxims
- Intuitive grasp of situations based on deep tacit understanding
- Analytic approaches only used in novel situations or when problems occur
- Has a vision of what is possible

Within their model, 'an expert generally knows what to do based upon mature and practiced understanding. . . . An expert's skill has become so much part of him that he need be no more aware of it than he is of his own body. . . . the expert manager, surgeon, nurse, lawyer or teacher is totally engaged in a skilful performance. When things are proceeding normally, experts don't solve problems and don't make decisions; they do what normally works'.

This description of the expert working almost on autopilot was formulated at a time when artificial intelligence was rapidly developing as a science. The Dreyfus brothers were keen to stress the differences between what would be possible with the purely logical approach that a computer could offer compared to the highly complex web of skills that need to be developed at expert level, many of them based upon tacit knowledge that cannot easily be expressed.

CLINICAL DECISION-MAKING

Rather than over-complicating the situation, the Dreyfus brothers may have oversimplified it. It is sobering to think that educational theorists still find it extremely difficult to pin down the precise process that so most of us go through many times each day.

We tend to take what we do when we consult for granted, and it is fascinating to consider just how complicated this process actually is. I am sure that upon reflection this hypothesis will strike a chord with many clinicians: we use our experience to quickly apply a filter to the cases that we see, but a good clinician will remain alert to any warning signs that a particular case does not fit into an expected pattern. An inexperienced clinician will have been taught much more of a 'building block' approach, stacking up all the blocks of evidence before trying to extract meaning from them. As they become more experienced, the threshold at which they do not need to go back to basics in order to reach a working diagnosis gradually increases.

It seems that experts swop between several different levels of cognition, depending upon the nature of the case that is presented to them. The Dreyfus model may well represent skilled behaviour under conditions of rapid interpretation and decision-making in which the separate processes of acquiring information, following routines, and making decisions become fully integrated, thanks to the accumulation of a vast set of memories of previous circumstance. Yet avoiding the pitfalls of jumping to false diagnoses requires more than that.

Research suggests that it is not the information base that a clinician holds that determines their level of expertise – in medicine this has been shown to peak when a doctor newly qualifies in a specialism. It also does not appear to be due to enhancement of deductive reasoning, as this is pretty much the same at graduation as later in the clinician's career, or it may even have a tendency to slightly decline. Rather, it seems that experts develop a complex set of patterns that have variously been described as templates, frames and scripts that contain a rich set of data about a particular illness and enables them to be recognized quickly. In experts, this is enhanced by memories of specific cases that highlight certain aspects of the disease.

There is sometimes also a need for an expert to recognize that a case does not fit one of the previously recognized scripts, and this ability to pick out the exceptional is clearly crucial, or mistakes will frequently be made. In those instances, the expert may need to return to a knowledge of the underlying physiological and pathological processes to try and fathom out the answers. The technique of problem-oriented medicine has been developed in recent years, and is being proposed as a diagnostic framework at all levels of expertise. It is likely that the cognitive response when an expert clinician is presented with a case will range across a continuum from intuitive as per the Dreyfus model, to analytical depending upon '...the complexity of the task, the ambiguity of content of the task, and the form of task presentation' (Hammond, et al. 1980),

Sue Shuttleworth (2006) considers the link between experience and consulting skills in her Doctoral thesis, and comes up with the following hypothesis:

'The advanced GP vet makes an intuitive decision based on all the different evidence available early on in the diagnostic process as to where in the continuum from healthy, to common condition to problem case that the tentative diagnosis is likely to be. Depending on this decision, the advanced GP vet will then tend to use an emergent pattern recognition followed by attempted falsification approach to confirm or deny a tentative diagnosis at the healthy end of this continuum, compared to a reductionist (scientific hypothesis) method approach to the "problem case"'.

What is also essential for the general practitioner is the ability to recognize when a case is beyond their expertise, and seek out more specialized advice for its care (Figure 7.1 illustrates a schematic representation of the clinical decision-making processes).

The Dreyfus model is also an attempt to identify the cognitive processes that are carried out at the various levels of ability, not necessarily what should be carried out. In particular, it allows little room for conscious reflection. It should not be assumed that those designated as experts are always correct, they are as prone to the fallibilities of human judgement as anyone else, and may in time allow their expertise to become jaded and out of date. Thus it is critical, as we shall see in the next chapter, for experts to retain critical control over the more intuitive parts of their abilities by regular reflection, self-critique and a disposition to learn from colleagues.

What Are the Key Skills that Practitioners Need to Develop?

The skills that practitioners require are often complex, calling not only for new information, but also for new ways of analysing, evaluating, interpreting and applying knowledge. For example, we are often required to synthesize our clinical and case management abilities with personnel management, teamwork and communication skills.

Research into artificial intelligence and knowledge elicitation among experts has strongly established a particularly interesting fact – people don't know what they know (Eraut, 1994). This came home strongly to me when I started out with my learning set of practitioners on my MSc, which was run by the Professional Development Foundation in conjunction with the National Centre for Work Based Learning at Middlesex University. As is now common with work-based learning, some of the credits towards the Award are given for APEL – the Accreditation of Prior Experiential Learning, which require the candidate to reflect upon selected aspects of their professional learning to date. We just couldn't get our heads around the concept of what we had learnt during the

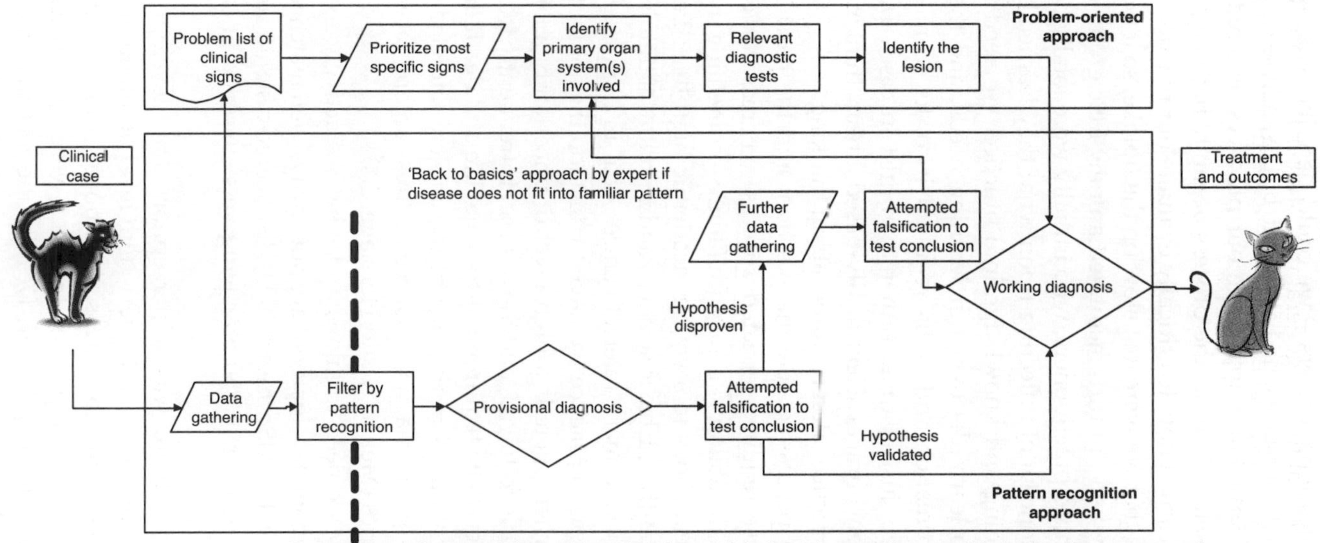
Problem-oriented approach
Problem list of clinical signs
Prioritize most specific signs
Identify primary organ system(s) involved
Relevant diagnostic tests
Identify the lesion
Clinical case
'Back to basics' approach by expert if disease does not fit into familiar pattern
Further data gathering
Attempted falsification to test conclusion
Treatment and outcomes
Working diagnosis
Hypothesis disproven
Data gathering
Filter by pattern recognition
Provisional diagnosis
Attempted falsification to test conclusion
Hypothesis validated
Pattern recognition approach

Students are usually taught to take a problem-oriented approach to diagnosis, generating a complete data base for every case and then working from basic principles. This technique is not generally used by an experienced general practitioner working under the normal time constraints, who are thought to keep a mesh of disease templates in their mind, which they match to cases. It is only if this system fails that an experienced practitioner will resort to a more systematic approach. The ability to 'expect the unexpected' and pick out cases that subtly fail to conform to a preconceived pattern is at least one important aspect of true expertise.

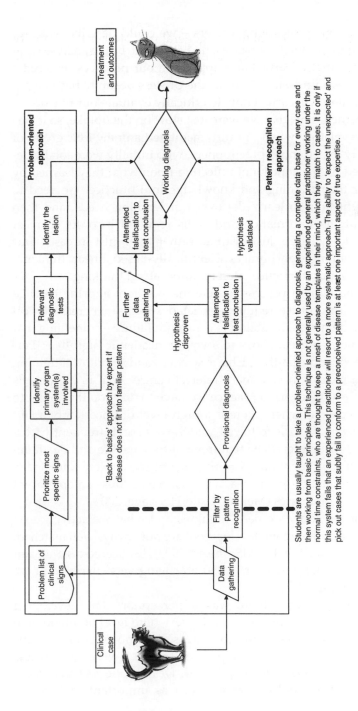

Figure 7.1 A flow chart of a model of the clinical decision-making process.

course of our professional careers – we could describe what we had done, and what courses we had attended, but to analyse what we had actually learned and applied in our practices required a whole new mindset. With time, the process began to become automatic, and we learned how to critically evaluate our practice.

It seemed to us that we were just slow on the uptake, so it was again revelatory when I in turn facilitated an new MSc group of similarly experienced practitioners, who initially were totally bewildered by the concept of reflecting upon what they learned by putting their training and knowledge into practice. We need to be taught how to learn, discover our learning needs, and then seek out the information and skills required in order to meet them – knowledge 'just in time' rather than 'just in case'. Our training strongly encourages scientifically-based 'linear' thinking, whereas clinical practice often requires lateral thinking.

The admission process to veterinary school and the passage through the course requires repeated success, whereas clinical practice demands the ability to cope with failure – something that can come as a great shock to a young, academic high-flyer. Perhaps most importantly, the basic sciences and the clinical training that we receive in veterinary referral centres deal in high levels of certainty, whereas in practice we have to develop the ability to make decisions where there is a high level of uncertainty about the correct path to be followed, and the data set is frequently frustratingly incomplete. The requirement to make life and death decisions about our patients in the face of incomplete knowledge and inadequate support is a major source of stress among recent veterinary graduates (Mellanby and Herrtage, 2004).

What we know we need to know, and what we actively seek out in our professional development are not always well matched. Sue Shuttleworth in her MSc thesis (2003) discovered a significant mismatch among more than 850 practicing vets surveyed in the UK (see Table 7.1).

Not surprisingly, there was a perception that developing clinical skills was important, and a very high level of intention to obtain further training in those areas. Additional surgical skills were not seen as being as important, but they were nevertheless the next most likely to be pursued. Despite the fact that client communication skills were not seen as important in terms of

Table 7.1

Skill Ranked in Importance	% Likelihood of Obtaining Them
1. Additional clinical skills	90%
2. Leadership skills	52%
3. Personal planning skills	27%
4. Time management skills	25%
5. Additional operating skills	69%
6. Computer skills	44%
7. Client communication skills	47%
8. Practice planning skills	46%

professional learning, they were still ranked fourth in terms of those most likely to be sought. The most glaring mismatch is in the areas of time management and personal planning skills, where respondents were perfectly well aware of how important they were to their professional career, yet seemingly had little intention of following up this perceived need with some extra training in those areas. Perhaps this is because of a lack of availability of such training, or a perception that they cannot effectively be taught, or maybe, most ironically of all, due to a lack of time!

When it comes to the development of our postgraduate learning, the most important message that this book can impart is that it's unlikely that the primary issue that will hamper you professional development will be a lack of clinical acumen. Whilst it is important to keep up to date with new knowledge and skills, this part of our professional learning seems to take pretty good care of itself. As a profession, we are highly motivated to develop these areas, at least in fields that interest us. Yet our clients generally take our clinical ability for granted, and where they do have doubts, are often very poorly placed to make any sort of objective judgement about our level of proficiency. The key areas are much more focused on the 'softer' clinical skills, such as our ability to convince our clients that we care about their animals, our ability to communicate with them effectively and our ability to convince them that what we are offering is value for money.

Some practitioners feel that an individual either has those skills or not, and those that do not will simply drift away from practice into other branches of the profession. We have already established in Chapter 5 that communication skills are not just a personality trait, but are a series of skills that can be learned, aided by the use of appropriate teaching methods.

Another widely held argument is that those skills cannot be taught, but simply develop with experience. The concept that experiential learning is intrinsic and inevitable is an attractive one, and to some extent there may be an element of truth in that assertion. However, if it were universally true, practitioners would become uniformly more proficient as they became more experienced. Figures from the Royal College of Veterinary Surgeons, the governing body of the veterinary profession in the UK, show that complaints from the public relating to professional competence are most common during the early stages of a career, and again towards the end (Preliminary Investigation Committee report to RCVS Council, June 2007). Experience and learning do not automatically follow on one from the other, and a great deal of work has been carried out to demonstrate that formalizing the process of linking the two can greatly enhance its effectiveness for most people.

How Can Practitioners Best Develop Their Expertise?

I hear and I forget; I see and I remember; I do and I understand. (Old Chinese proverb)

There are a wide variety of different means in which a practitioner can develop his or her learning, but he or she can be divided into three main categories:

Published Information

Scientific journals have traditionally been considered to be the most authoritative source of veterinary knowledge, and we have already discussed in Chapter 5 how recent years have seen an explosion in the number of journals that compete for our attention. *The Trouble with Medical Journals* (2006) by Richard Smith, the highly respected ex-editor of the *British Medical Journal*, makes salutary reading for anyone who wishes to take a critical look at the system which forms the bedrock of our scientific understanding. After reviewing the uncertainties and biases associated with the various scientific methodologies, he goes on to examine another Holy Grail of the system – peer review. It is ironic that a process that is designed to protect the scientific method is intrinsically so unscientific. He quotes several studies that the *British Medical Journal* carried out, where they deliberately inserted major errors into papers that they then sent out to many reviewers: nobody ever spotted all of the errors; some did not spot any, and on average around one quarter of the errors were picked up. It rarely uncovers fraud, because the whole system of scientific integrity works primarily upon trust. The inconsistencies in responses to papers sent out to multiple reviewers were marked. He quotes two reviewers commenting on the same paper:

Reviewer A: I found this paper an extremely muddled paper with a large number of deficits.

Reviewer B: It is written in a clear style and would be understood by any reader.

The concerns expressed in the book refer specifically to medical journals. The process for veterinary journals, that have a much smaller readership, may tend to be even less rigorous. A much more open system of peer review would add transparency to the process and remove the cloak of anonymity that some reviewers use to hide their biases and deficiencies, although it is argued that that would leave us without anyone to review the ever-increasing mountain of articles that are being submitted.

If we consider other forms of published information, the scope of bias and misinformation is even greater – text books rapidly fall out of date, and often rely upon 'eminence-based medicine' rather than advocating treatment based upon a careful examination of the evidence. The internet is increasingly being used to retrieve information, and can more easily be kept up to date, yet its source has to be checked carefully. For example, many commercial organizations use the internet to promote information that may be based upon scientific method, but is carefully selected to promote their own interests.

So, can we believe anything that we read? John Ioannidis (2005), a respected researcher from Greece, puts forward a convincing argument why 'most published research findings are false', so that if you spend your time reading medical journals, you may more often be misled than informed. But then, since it was a paper published in a scientific journal, we may feel free to treat its conclusions with scepticism. It is the scepticism that is important – we need to be constantly questioning the evidence put before us, or at the very least, encourage those that we trust to evaluate if for us.

Learning from Others

> If you have an apple and I have an apple and we exchange these apples then you and I will still have one apple. But if you have an idea and I have an idea and we exchange those ideas, then each of us will have two ideas. (George Bernard Shaw)

This category raises the question: 'Who is best placed to educate practicing veterinarians?' The existing paradigm for postgraduate veterinary education is very much based around academics telling practitioners what they think they need to know. There is no doubt that academics play a vital role in laying down the bedrock of scientific knowledge for our professional practice, but it must also be remembered that their approach to a clinical problem is likely to be driven by different priorities:

- An academic will be keen to understand a clinical case in order to gain further insight and knowledge. A practitioner is likely to be more orientated towards taking practical action to solve a problem.
- The cost and timescale of achieving a resolution to a problem are likely to be of much less concern to an academic than to a practitioner.
- Academics are usually informed by their own research, but by the experience of others, whereas practitioners are informed by the research of others but their own direct experience.
- The academic's ideal means of communication is generally written, with the long-term objective of publishing data, and

the demands of scholarship will tend to appeal to an introverted personality type. Practitioners are likely to prefer face-
to-face communication, where any objections and issues can
be raised and dealt with immediately, and will consequently
tend towards an extroverted personality type, more suited to
the art of verbal communication and persuasion.

- Academics deal with uncertainty by addressing it explicitly
and assigning statistical limits to it. The practitioner is almost
always in a more complex position, where a wide variety of
different sources of information, sometimes conflicting, will
need to be weighed up, and action taken on the basis of their
opinion, usually after discussing the options with their client.

These differences are not highlighted in an effort to argue that
one approach is superior to the other, simply because academics
and practitioners often work within different paradigms. The assumption that an individual well-versed in the scientific basis of
a particular specialty is necessarily the best person to encourage
professional learning among practitioners may be flawed. That is
not to say that there is never a need for practitioners to gain an
insight into the way in which such issues are dealt with within an
academic environment, but the door should also be left open for
other forms of professional learning that is based upon their own
work experience, and that of their peers.

So, how effective are Continuing Education (CE) courses at improving the way in which we practice? They are the traditional
answer to meeting our professional developmental requirements,
to the point where the mandatory CPD requirements for many
of the veterinary governing bodies depend upon proof of atten-
dance of a minimum number of hours. Unfortunately, all the evidence suggests that unless they are planned in order to meet specific learning needs, and their learning outcomes are followed up
promptly after a return to the workplace, they are one of the least
effective ways of improving performance.

A more effective means of learning within a social environment
is the establishment of peer learning groups of professionals with
a common objective. Such a group can offer mutual support for
a group faced with a shared problem, and techniques such as

brainstorming can be used to hammer out ideas and take them forwards. There are many tools such as SWOT analyses (strengths; weaknesses; opportunities and threats) to help provide a structure to the group learning process.

An extremely powerful tool to encourage group learning is **action learning** in a group of about six people that get together on a regular basis to deal with a common problem. In this context, a problem is specifically defined as an issue for which there is no existing solution, so that different people in different circumstances will propose different ways to resolve it. This is as opposed to a puzzle, which is considered to be an issue to which one specific answer exists. The people involved may be a cross-section of members of one practice, or they may be peers from different practices with a common aim, such as completing a postgraduate qualification. At least in the early stages, action learning sets require a trained facilitator to keep the proceedings on course, but that facilitator must play the role of an expert in the learning process, rather than providing expertise in the problem area being tackled.

So, what is the difference between an action learning group and any other peer group working towards a shared aim? Any such group needs to establish its own ground rules, which are always designed to provide a protected and confidential learning environment, where no individual is able to 'pull rank' on another. The essence of action learning is based around insightful questioning. The spirit is one of dialogue (a greater understanding through the shared word) rather than discussion, which involves a breaking-down of different views. The aim is not to 'win points' by promoting a particular point of view, but to encourage the member of the group airing a particular problem to think more deeply about the issues behind it, and thus come up with ways of solving it. This could involve going outside the group to seek additional propositional knowledge or technical skills.

Krystyna Weinstein (1999) lists the key outcomes that a good action learning programme can provide:

- Gaining new knowledge and information
- Reasoning differently

- Behaving differently
- Becoming more aware
- Gaining greater understanding of oneself and one's motives
- Altering beliefs and values
- Acknowledging feelings and their impact

It is obvious that this form of learning is an ideal way of developing the non-technical skills that we have already identified as being the key to good veterinary practice.

Practical Tips for CPD/CE

- Avoid attending CPD/CE events only because they take your fancy, are convenient, or free.
- Take some time to identify your learning needs and write them down for future reference.
- Translate those needs into learning objectives and carefully consider how you could best achieve them.
- Set yourself clear targets and timescales so that that you can measure your success in meeting them. In some instances you may even wish to measure this in financial terms, so that you can estimate the cost effectiveness of your learning.
- Structure your CPD/CE to meet those needs. Think outside the traditional box of attending courses: there may be other ways of more effectively gaining the knowledge and skills that you require.
- Consider how you will follow up your learning to ensure that it results in lasting changes to the way you perform in your work. New knowledge needs to be repeatedly applied in order to reinforce its effect.
- Reflect back upon your CPD/CE at regular intervals, reviewing how closely it has helped you to meet your objectives. Ask yourself if the objectives need to be re-framed.

This structured approach to CPD/CE will not only help to guide your own professional development, but can be used as a framework if you are required to appraise the development of other members of your practice team, at whatever level.

Experiential Learning

There has been a great deal of research into the nature of experiential learning and its effectiveness. One of the most useful definitions is provided by McGill and Warner Weil (1989), who see it as

> *The process whereby people individually and in association with others, engage in direct encounter, then* purposefully *reflect upon, validate, transform, give personal meaning to and seek to integrate their different ways of knowing. Experiential learning therefore enables the discovery of possibilities that may not be evident from direct alone.*

Experience needs to be consciously processed in order to for knowledge to result from it, and that requires a certain degree of effort and to be instigated with a specific desire to learn.

Reflective practice is vital to this process, and so the next chapter is dedicated to that process, but for the moment I would like to consider how we can enhance the way in which we learn from our experience.

Neighbour (2005) stresses the benefits of awareness-based learning rather than instruction-based teaching. When mentoring others (and the same concept can be applied when reflecting upon our own actions), he suggests that we should take a questioning approach:

What?
- Do you think about this?
- What do you mean by. . .?

Where?
- Where is your focus of attention at the current point?

When?
- When did you notice. . .?
- What was the sequence of events. . .?

How?
- How do you know that is the case?
- How can you tell?
- By what process does it come about?
- How happy are you about this?

Why? – elicits values and beliefs
- Why did you choose that drug?
- Why did you opt for…?
- Why not consider…?
- What principles are involved here…?
- What is your opinion about…?

The nature of the questions that Neighbour has listed are very similar to the type of insightful questions that members of a learning set would pose to someone trying to solve a problem. This is no coincidence, as the encouragement of reflection upon our work practices is a major aim of action learning. A similar questioning approach can be used within the context of a one-to-one tutoring relationship, so that it becomes a form of coaching rather than teaching.

13 Tips to Help You Learn (after Honey and Mumford, 1993)

1. Identify your own learning needs
2. Establish effective criteria as learning objectives
3. Measure how effective you are (see exercise below)
4. Produce your own personalized learning plan
5. Take advantage of learning opportunities in your practice
6. Review your progress regularly
7. Listen to what others have to say about your learning needs and progress
8. Accept help when it is offered
9. Face up honestly to unwelcome information about your learning deficiencies
10. Take risks and tolerate anxieties
11. Analyse what other successful practitioners do
12. Know yourself
13. Share information

Exercise – Structuring CPD/CE

Draw up a competency profile of the skills that you consider that you need for your job. In order to do that, you might like to start with the list of skills in the table on page 149, and then break them down further. Then rate yourself against each of those skills on a scale of one to ten – you could extend this to a 360° profile by asking other members of your practice team to score you on the same basis.

This profile should then enable you to highlight any particularly weak areas of competence that you need to develop. Consider carefully how you could most effectively improve your performance in one of those areas and formulate a six-month programme to develop your learning in that area. Consider also how you will be able to reassess your competence in that area at the end of that period in the most objective manner possible – perhaps by repeating a 360° assessment. At the end of the period, write down a short reflection upon the learning process, how well you feel you have reached your objective, and how you can continue to take the process forwards.

THE GENERATION OF NEW KNOWLEDGE FROM PRACTICE

I have already mentioned how the application of propositional knowledge to an individual case in itself creates new knowledge, but because of the nature of this knowledge it is usually not recorded and so has to be learnt time and time again. We are accustomed to the paradigm where research is generated in academic institutions and handed down to practitioners to develop, but there is a growing recognition within human medicine of the value of collating and analysing research data at grass roots level for dissemination outwards to other practitioners.

The nature of the data collected in these two different ways may tend to differ. That collated within a research environment will often be more highly quantitative and 'scientific'. Those results can be more confidently generalized to other cases, providing that they are selected from a similar sample of the population. The weakness is that that cross-section may be skewed by the data that an external researcher will be able to sample.

A practitioner is likely to be able to collate research data from cases that are more relevant to the typical scenario seen in practice, but is less likely to be able to record the volume of data in order to produce the same confidence in the generalizability of the results. Yet the more qualitative data may still be invaluable in terms of alerting other practitioners to the more subtle nuances that are seen in individual cases, and in turn perhaps trigger more quantitative research.

In a classic confrontation, a scientist might say

If you can't count it, it's not worth knowing.

However, a practice-based researcher with a more qualitative bent may counter that with:

If you can count it, then it's probably not 'it'.

The truth is that both quantitative and qualitative research methodologies potentially have a lot to offer the profession, but they tell us different things in different ways. The important parameter is that whichever underlying methodology is used, it is rigorously applied to validate the data, and that the findings are then interpreted with an understanding of the strengths and weaknesses of the methodologies used. What cannot be doubted is that there is an urgent need both for more first-opinion data to be collated by practitioners, and for more clinical research to be carried out in academic institutions. The former often helps us to answer 'What questions should we be asking?', and the latter will then help to answer those questions.

SUMMARY

This chapter began with the premise that learning is the key to a successful career in veterinary practice. This is not a new concept, as it is over 2400 years since Socrates declared:

An unquestioning life is not worth living.

Once we begin to reflect upon the nature of professional expertise, we can see that it involves a great deal more than just the assembly of building blocks of information that can be re-assembled to solve the problems that we face in our workplace, although such information does have its place. The undergraduate veterinary course demands that students develop the ability to soak up and regurgitate vast amounts of information. There is a move towards a more cognitive and less didactic approach to the undergraduate course, but the majority of us within the profession have not 'learnt how to learn', and so have developed those essential skills in a very haphazard way.

As a profession, we still see the acquisition of additional clinical skills as the most important aim of our professional development. Although we recognize that a whole range of ancillary skills are of crucial importance to the effectiveness with which we are able to deliver care to our clients and our patients, we are nevertheless still reluctant to put effort into enhancing them. To some extent, that may be because we are unsure how to go about it, or even unconvinced that it is possible.

When it comes to pursuing an effective programme of professional development, we need to ensure that we take a strategic approach to our learning, which first involves honestly and accurately assessing our learning needs. This involves reflection upon our practice, which is dealt with in the following chapter. We then need to assess what form of learning will best meet those needs – a very different approach to just booking in to CPD/CE courses that take our fancy.

When assessing the forms of learning that are available to us, we need to keep our personal learning objectives in mind, as well as an understanding of our own learning styles. This enables us to select a programme of learning that is likely to be truly transformational and so benefit our work.

One fundamental tenet of professional learning is being able to maintain a tolerable but motivating level of self-questioning; a healthy scepticism that leads to an enquiring mind that questions many of the everyday assumptions that we make. Being excessively smug and complacent in our working environment can be self-deluding and dangerous, and a mild degree of 'constructive discomfort' can provide a source of tension that stimulates us to overcome our inherent tendency to accept everything at face value. Constantly questioning the validity of everything that we do can rapidly become self-destructive, so this advice needs to be tempered with a dose of common sense, but we should bear in mind that when things feel *too* comfortable, we are probably not challenging and stretching our abilities as far as we should.

We therefore need to recognize that there are many external factors that cause bias within the published material that is available to us, and that even the information in peer-reviewed professional journals has to be reviewed critically. Whilst the experience of others, particularly those that specialize in a particular clinical field, may be of relevance to us, we also need to evaluate their information critically, and consider whether it is based upon evidence or eminence. Attending a course is only likely to be of significant benefit to our performance in the workplace if it is carefully selected to meet our recognized learning needs, and followed up quickly by work-based application and reflection to reinforce it.

Whilst we tend to overestimate the value of formalized courses, we greatly underestimate the benefit of structured experiential work-based learning. Although we know that we gather experience as we practice, it is only when we reflect upon that experience in a formal way that we can maximize our learning, and discover those areas where we most need to develop our knowledge and skills. This can be done on a personal level, or via e-learning, but the power of a group of peers to come together to mutually enhance their professional learning, preferably with the assistance of an experienced facilitator, should not be underestimated.

A great deal of new knowledge can be generated from general practice in this way, but most of it is lost to the profession because it is not analysed and recorded. The nature of this knowledge may be different to the more quantitative data that can be generated by large-scale research projects from within centres of research, but because it is generated from first opinion work and is grounded in practice, it is different but not necessarily inferior. A great deal of more qualitative and quantitative research is now being carried out from within human primary care, and projects such as the outreach programme being run by Dr Mark Holmes at the Cambridge Infectious Diseases Consortium (see http://www.vet.cam.ac.uk/cidc/training/outreach.html) which use government funding to help train practitioners in methodologies of clinical research and encourage their work, signal a way forward within the veterinary profession.

If you just want to read one book...

Michael Eraut's book was published in 1994, but the concepts within it are still highly relevant, and it provides a sound understand of the nature of professional knowledge and how it can be developed.

Eraut, M. (1994). *Developing Professional Knowledge and Competence*. London: RoutledgeFalmer.

Should you just wish to find out more about action learning, and understand more about what this powerful synergistic process can be harnessed, Krystna Weinstein's little book on the subject makes easy and fascinating reading.

Weinstein, K. (1999). *Action Learning – a Practical Guide*, 2nd edn. Aldershot: Gower.

The Reflective Practitioner

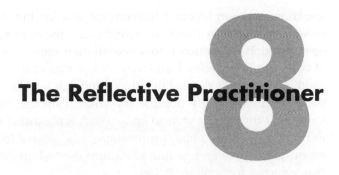

Presenting the argument that reflective practice is a valuable tool for professional development is the main task. (Charalambous, 2003)*

It was with considerably thought (or dare I say, reflection) that I decided to make this topic a chapter in its own right. Firstly, it is so closely interwoven with the previous chapter on postgraduate education that it has been a challenge to decide how to separate the topics. Secondly, my experience of the reaction from the veterinary profession to the term 'reflective practice' has been

* Charalambous, A. (2003). Reflective practice as a facilitator for learning. *Icus Nurse Web Journal*, Issue 13 January–March 2003. http://www.nursing.gr/reflectiveprac.pdf. Reprinted with permission.

less than positive. Mention the concept to a teacher, or a health professional such as a nurse or a medic, and they embrace it with open arms. But mention it to a veterinarian more than a couple of years out of vet school, and they look at you as if you are from another planet. It's not just that they often don't understand what the term means. They don't know what it means, but they *do* know that they don't *want* to know what it means! It all sounds too touchy-feely for a busy professional, who is used to rolling up his or her sleeves and getting stuck into the task in hand, rather than pausing for contemplation.

But that is precisely why I have decided that the issue of reflective practice is so important that it deserves its place as the penultimate chapter of my book. If there is one concept that encapsulates the most effective way to continuously learn in the workplace, this is it.

WHAT IS REFLECTIVE PRACTICE?

Reflection in general is a form of mental processing that we apply to relatively ill-structured and complex problems for which there is no obvious single solution. It is largely based upon a further processing of knowledge and understanding that we already possess. Within an academic context, it needs to be formalized, with a conscious and stated purpose for the process. It is normally processed into either a written or verbalized form for others to consider and possibly to assess.

Reflective practice helps us to:

- Understand what we already know. We all start from our own position of knowledge and have our own set of experiences from which to draw.
- Identify what we need to know in order to advance understanding of the subject. Professional learning does not operate in a vacuum but in the context of our work.
- Make sense of new information and feedback in relation to our own experience.
- Guide choices for further learning. Having made sense of new information and integrated it into an existing framework of

understanding, it is then possible to make informed choices of what to do next and how to develop our understanding.
- To develop appropriate learning behaviour, such as by slowing down the pace of learning to provide 'intellectual space', developing a sense of personal ownership of the learning process, and improving the emotional intelligence that enables us to understand our own learning processes (known as metacognition).

Donald Schön (1983) first suggested that the capacity to reflect on action so as to engage in a process of continuous learning was one of the defining characteristics of professional practice. He argued that the model of professional training which he termed 'Technical Rationality' – of charging students up with knowledge in training schools so that they could discharge when they entered the world of practice, akin to the 'brick wall' approach to learning discussed in the previous chapter – has never been a particularly good description of how professionals 'think in action', and is quite inappropriate to practice in a fast-changing world. He described the four stages of the experiential learning cycle (see Figure 8.1).

This feedback loop can continue, because as we reflect upon what has happened after an intervention, we may well think about a further intervention that might facilitate the process, such as a follow-up phone call from a nurse if the appointment for the blood test has not been made within a specified time. Those of us who think we carry out everything we do optimally are seriously deluded, and within a learning organization everyone should be examining critically what they do and working out how to do it more effectively. Contrast this with a more didactic form of learning, where we may be told by an expert about how best to approach a case, and we then attempt to apply it to our work – the reality is that that approach very rarely results in a change in the way in which we carry out our work.

The cultivation of the capacity to reflect in action (while doing something) and on action (after you have done it) has now been accepted as an important feature of professional training in many disciplines. The cycle can begin at any stage, and it is interesting to see how these four stages of the experiential learning cycle fit

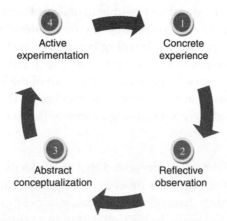

To take an example from practice:

1. I suggest to a client with a nephritic cat that they should have a blood test and blood pressure check to monitor their cat's condition, but the client refuses on the grounds that the cat now seems well and further intervention seems unnecessary.

2. After the event, I reflect upon why I did not achieve what I aimed to do. Why did I not convince the client that it was necessary? Am I sufficiently convinced about the need for monitoring of such cases?

3. I theorize that I need to be more convinced about the benefits of the routine monitoring of nephritic patients, and look up some clinical information on the management of the condition. I decide that a handout to reinforce the message may be useful.

4. I produce a handout on the monitoring of nephritic cats. The exercise has also made me clearer in my mind about why it is beneficial to the patient and may help prevent sudden (and potentially costly) complications. The next time I re-check a nephritic cat I am much more positive about what needs to be done, and have the information to back up my advice.

Figure 8.1 Experiential learning cycle.

in with the four learning styles described by Honey and Mumford (1982) (see Figure 8.2).

Each of us will have a bias towards one particular style of learning – and likewise, teachers will tend to be biased towards a particular approach. In order for the learning process to be optimized, it is necessary to correct any bias to obtain balance, which enables the whole cycle to be completed, and ideally repeated as a positive feedback loop. For example, pure scientists will tend to be much

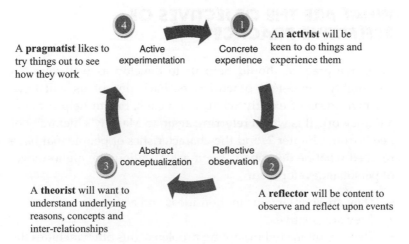

Figure 8.2   Learning styles.

stronger in abstract conceptualization of a problem, but need to consider the practicalities of its application. Conversely, someone working in a very practical environment where they often have to use their intuition to react to a situation (and this often applies within veterinary general practice) will tend towards a more pragmatic/activist approach, and therefore needs to ensure that they take time to reflect upon their activities and theorize about their relevance. An 'all-round learner' will have the balance to be able to manage all stages of this process effectively.

IS REFLECTIVE PRACTICE THE SAME AS EXPERIENTIAL LEARNING?

The two concepts are obviously closely related, but experiential learning will by definition involve some external experience. It will also usually involve reflection, unless the material of learning is so unchallenging to the learner that reflection is unnecessary. Reflective practice does not necessarily have to involve a novel external experience (although it usually does), as it can be a form of 'cognitive housekeeping' where internal experiences are the subject of the reflective process that is then applied in the workplace.

WHAT ARE THE OBJECTIVES OF REFLECTIVE PRACTICE?

Reflective practice should help us to develop as well-rounded and highly competent practitioners. Each one of us will have our own ideas of exactly what that means, but to help provide a framework, it is worth referring again to Maslow's hierarchy of needs from Chapter 2, and the characteristics of people that have reached what he described as self-actualization, the highest level of personal development:

- They are spontaneous in their ideas and actions.
- They are creative.
- They are interested in solving problems; this often includes the problems of others. Solving these problems is often a key focus in their lives.
- They feel a closeness to other people, and generally appreciate life.
- They have a system of morality that is fully internalized and independent of external authority.
- They have discernment and are able to view all things in an objective manner.

More specifically within the context of our professional work, we can look for several indicators of such development:

- Complexity and differentiation – the ability to hand diverse and unfamiliar situations.
- Organization and integration – the ability to make sense of a complex situation and connect various seemingly separate elements.
- Flexibility – the ability to respond in different ways, depending upon the situation.
- Sensitivity – being aware of details and nuances.
- Mobility and dynamics – such as curiosity and openness to new situations and ideas.
- Internal control – the ability to delay self-gratification for the long-term good.
- Efficiency – in the manner in which one uses the resources available to reach one's goals.

It is also useful to look at the descriptors that have been laid down by the RCVS in the UK for candidates taking their new modular postgraduate certificate (see www.rcvs.org.uk/modcerts). They are based upon generic descriptors developed by the Quality Assurance Agency that outline the level of understanding expected from candidates completing a master's degree in the UK and outline the nature of the cognitive processes that an advanced practitioner should be applying to their work.

Candidates will need to demonstrate:
- A thorough understanding of the knowledge base, including latest developments within the subject area of professional veterinary practice and postgraduate education opportunities for work-based learning.
- Originality in the application, creation and interpretation of knowledge within veterinary professional practice.
- Conceptual understanding that enables them to:
  - o Evaluate critically current literature and research with regard to professional practice.
  - o Develop a critique and if appropriate propose new approaches to their personal professional practice.

Typically, holders of the qualification will be able to:
- Deal with complex issues in an organized and creative manner, make sound judgements in the absence of complete data, and communicate their conclusions clearly to veterinary colleagues and to non-veterinary audiences, including clients.
- Demonstrate self-direction and originality in tackling and solving problems, and act autonomously in planning and implementing tasks in their professional area of work.
- Continue to advance their knowledge and understanding, and to develop new skills to a high level.

They will have the qualities and transferable skills necessary for professional veterinary work requiring:
- The exercise of initiative and personal responsibility
- Decision-making in complex and unpredictable situations
- The independent learning ability required for CPD

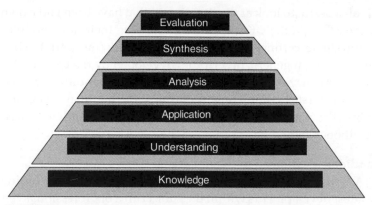

Knowledge:
arrange, define, duplicate, label, list, memorize, name, order, recognize, relate, recall, repeat, reproduce
Understanding:
classify, describe, discuss, explain, express, identify, indicate, locate, recognize, report, restate, review, select, translate
Application:
apply, choose, demonstrate, dramatize, employ, illustrate, interpret, operate, practice, schedule, sketch, solve, use, write
Analysis:
analyse, appraise, calculate, categorize, compare, contrast, criticise, differentiate, distinguish, examine, experiment, question, test
Synthesis:
arrange, assemble, collect, compose, construct, create, design, develop, formulate, manage, organize, plan, prepare, propose, set up, write
Evaluation:
appraise, argue, assess, attach, choose, compare, defend, estimate, judge, predict, rate, select, support, value, evaluate, core

Figure 8.3   Bloom's taxonomy of thinking skills.

Finally, it is worth considering Bloom's taxonomy of thinking skills (see Figure 8.3), which has already been proposed as a framework to encourage a more advanced approach to the clinical diagnostic process (Nkanginieme, 1997). It starts with basic knowledge about a problem and moves up through deeper levels of thought, until it gets to synthesis and finally evaluation, where new knowledge is being created and its relative importance quantified. The words listed underneath each term are those that would be used to prompt that level of cognition.

Examples of questions that you could ask yourself about a problem to encourage synthesis would be:

- Can I see a possible solution to . . .?
- If I had access to all resources how would I deal with . . .?

- Can I develop a proposal that would . . .?
- How many ways can I . . .?
- Can I design a . . .?
- What would happen if I . . .?
- Devise my own way to deal with . . .?

and for evaluation:

- Is there a better solution to . . .?
- Judge the value of . . .?
- Can I defend my position about . . .?
- Do I think . . . is a good or bad thing?
- How would I have handled . . .?
- What changes to . . . would I recommend?
- How would I feel if . . .?
- How effective are . . .?
- What do I think about . . .?

All these indicators are inherent within the concept of an experienced, reflective practitioner, to which I would add one more: the ability to recognize and sensibly act upon tacit rather than explicit knowledge. The concept of tacit understanding of knowledge is an interesting one, and links with the idea of implicit learning and intuition. Daniel Goleman (2007) reviews the neuroscience behind the way in which the human brain stores and processes knowledge. Conscious cognition and quick decisions are made within the frontal lobes of the cerebral cortex, but lower portions of the brain such as the basal ganglia and the amygdale store emotions associated with memories. Implicit knowledge that we build up through our working lives is stored in this area, where learning occurs much more slowly than in the higher regions of the brain, but this may be where wisdom can be said to lie – the gut feeling that something feels right – a very special blend of cognition and emotion. The danger is that either we fail to recognize the knowledge that we have accumulated, or we fail to untangle it from the emotional entanglement within our more primitive learning centres. Reflective practice enables us to bring this type of knowledge to the forefront of our minds and consciously interpret it.

Reflective Writing

One of the major obstacles to the learning process is that practitioners fail to appreciate that whilst we all reflect upon our experiences at times, this is very different to the formal process of reflective practice. There are well-recognized stages in the depth of reflection that learners are able to practice as they progress, and that the act of expressing this externally, either in writing or verbally to other interested parties, in itself provide extra levels of learning because we have to modify ideas in order to represent them. Recording it in the written form of a reflective diary also enables us to refer back to it, and so reflect further upon developments that may have occurred with the passage of time, either externally due to new events, or internally due to our changing ability to interpret the information. This is best illustrated by taking three examples.

Consider each of the following short pieces that describe and reflect upon the same event to varying degrees. After reading each, jot down what your feel about the depth of reflection involved in each, and the characteristics that define it. Then compare your notes with those that I have appended about each piece at the end.

Managing Diabetes Mellitus in a Cat (1)

I saw an elderly cat with diabetes mellitus (DM) the other day. It was a busy evening surgery and I was struggling to keep up with the appointments, when an elderly lady brought in her 11-year-old cat with all the classical signs – polydipsia, a period of polyphagia, followed by loss of appetite and weight loss. By the time she brought him in he was a pretty sick cat, so I immediately took a small blood sample and ran a blood glucose. When that came up high, I was able to take a urine sample directly by cystocentesis, because his bladder was pretty full. I quickly discovered that not only his urine glucose but also his urine ketone levels were reading maximum on the dipstick.

I was pleased that I had been able to reach a diagnosis so promptly, and reported back to the owner that her cat had diabetes, was in a pretty bad way, but could be treated. I suggested that we keep the cat in overnight on a drip, start him immediately on soluble insulin, and then try to stabilize him so that he could go home on twice-daily injections.

It was obvious that the owner was very shocked at this diagnosis, although she must have been expecting something pretty seriously wrong with the cat, considering the state that he had deteriorated to. She enquired about the cost, and I explained that I could only give her a very rough estimate of the immediate care her cat needed, and that the ongoing costs of insulin, syringes etc. would not be too excessive. When I totted up the cost of the immediate intensive care for the first week of treatment, she said that there was no way she could afford that, he was an elderly, sick cat, and she would like him euthanized. I tried to explain that there was a strong chance that he would return to good health once we got his condition under control, and that the regular insulin injections were more easily managed than most people expected. I tried to assuage her concerns about cost by offering to come to some sort of arrangement so that she could pay off for his treatment over a period of time, or that we could even try and get some funding from the local branch of the RSPCA.

I felt that she just wasn't listening to what I was saying. It seemed as if she had made up her mind whilst I had been running the tests, or even before she arrived at the clinic, and she insisted that she did not want to embark on a costly course of treatment. I was in a real quandary – professionally I was very unhappy about putting the cat down, but I just felt that if I pushed her into treating the cat it would turn out to be one of those cases that just didn't do well. I was also under increasing time pressure, with appointments building up in the waiting room, so I hastily and somewhat gruffly agreed. I got her to sign a consent form, and very efficiently and somewhat coldly euthanized the cat. The owner burst into tears when her pet stopped breathing, thanked me profusely, and quickly left the surgery. I have been thinking about what happened since then, and feel really bad about the outcome, but I'm not sure what else I could have done.

Managing Diabetes Mellitus in a Cat (2)

I saw an elderly cat with DM the other day. It was a busy evening surgery and I was struggling to keep up with the appointments, when an elderly lady brought in her 11-year-old cat with all the classical signs. By the time she brought him in he was a pretty sick cat and I felt something needed to be done there and then, so I took a small blood sample and ran a blood glucose, and confirmed the diagnosis with a urine sample taken by cystocentesis.

I feel I did a really good job by recognizing the condition and confirming the diagnosis so promptly, and so I think I took it pretty personally when it turned out that the owner did not want it treated. I was upset that she did not seem to care enough about the cat to at least give treatment a chance, even though I made every effort to find a way to assist with the costs that were involved. I was also both irritated and anxious by the fact that this all happened in the middle of a busy evening surgery, and felt that if she had already made her mind up to put the cat to sleep, she should have said that at the outset.

Because of this, I think I let my emotional state impinge upon my professional behaviour. I felt I wanted to 'punish' the owner by making it clear when I euthanized her cat that it was against my better judgement. I carried it out efficiently but very coldly. This has left me feeling really bad, firstly because I think it is wrong to allow my personal emotions to affect the way I behave, and secondly because it did seem after the event that she was genuinely upset. Losing a pet is hard enough, and I had no right to try and make her suffer more than was necessary.

Managing Diabetes Mellitus in a Cat (3)

I have spent quite a bit of time over the past few days considering how I handled the euthanasia of an elderly cat with DM. The elderly owner had waited until it was quite acutely ill before bringing it in. She had seemed detached, but her reaction after I euthanized the cat made me realize that she had all sorts of anxieties related to her cat's condition, particularly cost, and I feel sure she was very fond of the cat.

Clinically, I consider I handled the case very well, diagnosing it promptly despite being in the middle of a busy evening surgery. I wondered afterwards if it would have been better to admit the cat and allow the diagnosis and its consequences to be broken to the owner more slowly. The decision to carry out euthanasia was made in haste, because the owner was concerned about starting to rack up an unmanageable bill, and I was feeling pressurized by the number of clients building up in the waiting room. At the time, I was upset about the case partly because I felt my excellent clinical diagnostics had been unappreciated, and because she did not have sufficient confidence in my abilities to believe that I would probably have been able to get the cat on the road to recovery without the costs becoming excessive. I had felt particularly bad after the event because I was very cold when I euthanized the cat, and that subconsciously I wanted to punish her for her decision.

I have since discussed the case with some colleagues, and they have pointed out that I might have avoided problems by discussing the various diagnostic and likely treatment options before I dived in head first and ran the tests. I do need to be more empathetic to an owner's perception of a situation and try to work out a mutually acceptable treatment plan rather than just rushing in with what I think is best for the patient, particularly when I am feeling stressed and under pressure. It has helped me to appreciate that not everyone deals with a sick pet in the same way as I would. For example, some owners are simply not happy about putting their pet through intensive treatment with an uncertain future, or keeping a pet alive on long-term medication. I need to realize that just because that is not in accordance with my own values, it does not mean that the owner of the pet (who is the one who has to administer and pay for the long-term care) has no right to their own point of view, and it does not necessarily mean that they value their pet any less than I would my own. In retrospect, I can think of many cases where the decision to euthanize a pet early rather than treat it would have turned out to be the best option for the animal concerned. That does not mean that I will necessarily agree to euthanize pets with treatable diseases any earlier than I would have previously, but that I will need to look at my strategy for handling such cases so that, when necessary, I can engineer the time to discuss the issues involved thoroughly with an owner.

A lot of learning from this episode has related to emotional intelligence. I am coming to realize that I need to be more actively conscious of my own emotions in a situation such as this, so that I can manage them more effectively. I also need to be more empathetic to the emotions of owners whose value systems are not necessarily identical to my own. This may then modify the way in which I react to them, but might also give me a better understanding on how in future I can best try and work towards an outcome that is more mutually acceptable to both parties. I understand that Daniel Goleman's book contains a great deal of useful information on this topic, and have resolved to order it from the library to read next week.

Time for the Post-Mortem   So, how do these three accounts of the same event compare in terms of style, and more importantly, in terms of the depth of reflection that they contain? I hope it is obvious that it increases significantly from example 1to 3, but I shall try to illustrate specifically why:

Version 1 relates what has occurred. There is some reference to the author's emotional reaction to events, but the role that those emotions may have had upon his actions is not explored. It is written entirely from the perspective of the author, with almost no reference to what the client might have been feeling. The account is related strictly chronologically as part of a narrative, and there is no focus upon the key events. There is a focus upon the clinical information and the author's clinical competence, but this is not at the heart of the issue involved in this particular case. It ends leaving the reader feeling that the author has gained no real insight into what went wrong, let alone how to prevent it happening in future. It is a largely descriptive account containing very little reflection upon the author's actions, and is the sort of account that someone is likely to produce when they first embark upon reflective writing.

Version 2 describes the same events, although it is significantly shorter as it does not contain as much clinical narrative. It does begin to raise the issues that were at the heart of the problems with this consultation, although they are only described as relating to the author, without giving much thought to the third party. The author is self-critical, which does demonstrate that he is standing back from events to some extent, to enable him to analyse what was going on. There is little evidence of experiential learning from the episode that would lead the reader to think that the scenario would be unlikely to repeat itself.

Version 3 is very different, and although the direct narrative is much more succinct, the greater depth of reflection does take up more space. The following points should lead the reader to conclude that some deep reflection and learning has taken place following the incident:

- There is textual evidence of the author standing back from himself after the event and trying to look at his behaviour objectively.
- The reflection is self-critical and questions the beliefs and values upon which the author's behaviour is based.
- The author is now giving a lot of thought to the viewpoint of the owner, and appreciating that there may be valid, or at least understandable, value systems that are different to his own.
- There is a realization that his actions were contextual at that time, and would be likely to vary depending upon other external factors, even given the same clinical conundrum.
- There is evidence that he has not only reflected upon the case in isolation, but has widened the discussion to include other trusted colleagues, and reflected further upon the feedback that was received.
- The author has reflected upon the learning process that he had gone through – this learning about the learning journey that one has passed through brings in a higher level of reflection known as metacognition.
- He has not only identified the key issues relating to emotional intelligence that could impact on his behaviour in such circumstances in future, but has also pinpointed some further learning that might then be applied in future.

If you have found this illustration of the differing depths of reflective practice enlightening, you may wish to take it a step further, by selecting a challenging situation that you have experienced in your own workplace and then writing up your own commentary on it at three different levels, similar to above. By committing pen to paper it will make you think more about the behaviours that indicate deeper levels of reflection. When you reflect back upon that learning experience, you may also better appreciate how the active process of written reflection usually impacts upon the learning process much more deeply than simply mulling it over in your mind.

I hope the previous examples have helped to illustrate how, with practice, your reflective practice can become increasingly insightful rather than descriptive. The process is a very personal one that each of us has to develop in our own way – to start with, just getting used to using the first person rather than the third can be challenging for a scientist trained to be dispassionate. Yet emotions are a vital part of our interpersonal communications, and we also need to recognize how our emotions can influence our own learning process (see Chapter 2 for more information on emotional intelligence). One of the strengths of learning in this way is that we develop a sense of empowerment and ownership of our professional development – it is something we can actively develop ourselves as we recognize our own learning needs and find ways to meet them, rather than something we passively receive. It stands in its own right, but should the need arise, we can also use our written notes as evidence that can be externally validated.

A key characteristic of deep reflection is that it recognizes the way in which knowledge is constructed by individuals piecing together information in their own personal way. This means that the same event can be seen in different ways by different people and that more often than not there are multiple versions of the same truth. The same person can conceive the same event differently if other circumstances that affect their attitude have changed. This requires the learner to develop the ability to stand back from themselves and view events from different viewpoints, often setting up an internal dialogue that questions their own motivation and behaviour.

LEARNING JOURNALS

These documents are almost certain to form part of an assessment portfolio for any work-based learning programmes, but it is really worth having a go at keeping one to encourage your reflective practice. You should experiment to find the format that works best for you, but anything that encourages you to go back over your diary and reflect back upon them again at a later date will help to develop your deep reflective skills.

Moon (2004) suggests you keep the following three sections, with any new learning highlighted in some way:

1. Everyday writing – not necessarily literally every day, but whenever you feel able to reflect upon the events of a day, particularly any provisional learning that has occurred. You need to make entries frequently enough to keep some sense of continuity to document.
2. Timespells – this accounts for the fact that periods of our lives appear to pass in 'chunks' – periods of stability interspersed by periods of change. The characteristics of each period are decided by the learner in retrospect, and the writing is more about the feelings that the events during each period inspired, rather than the events themselves. Someone with a more visual pattern of learning may find it easier to express these feelings in the form of a sketch, cartoon or a mind map rather than words. Entries in the Timespells section should be cross-referenced to the straightforward reflective writing in section 1.
3. Workings – a section for any writing that does not relate to a specific time period, but reflections that are inspired by internal thoughts and dialogues.

Start with everyday writing and see what format works best for you. You should find that returning to earlier reflections in the light of further experience will almost always provide further enlightenment, whatever structure you use. Jenny Moon suggests that 'Sometimes there is a struggle to make time to reflect. Make an appointment with yourself in your diary'.

SUMMARY

This chapter has brought together many of the strands within this book to consider the concept of reflective practice. I hope it has convinced you; it is very different to just 'thinking about something', and that the concept is highly relevant to producing success in veterinary practice, at whatever level we function. Anyone taking a postgraduate level qualification, in whatever area, will need to recognize firstly the personal traits that characterize an individual who aspires to such recognition, and then more specifically, the nature of their work that demonstrates their advanced capabilities. It is vital to grasp that a higher level of qualification should involve a greater depth of understanding and not just a larger amount of knowledge.

If striving towards a further qualification fits in with your goals, then you may find a good work-based higher degree to be an excellent framework to encourage your development, and should also provide external support to help develop those cognitive skills I have outlined. However, that route is not for everyone, but I would contend that every self-respecting veterinarian should pay attention to his or her standard of work, even if external validation is not formally required. Sue Shuttleworth (2006) gave this a great deal of thought in her doctoral thesis, and came up with the following three skills that veterinary professionals need to develop in order to self-validate their professional development:

- **Self-audit** is an important competency for the professional. It is essential though that this is carried out at a level that is appropriate for the individual, taking into consideration experiences to date, the work being carried out and the personal, employers and professional values and beliefs. This allows an ongoing and realistic assessment to be made of the quality of the professional work carried out by an individual.
- **Self-directed learning** ensures that the professional considers all aspects of their learning requirements, not just those that they find more interesting. They actively seek out learning

opportunities, and find these from often unexpected events. The act of learning becomes important and explicit.

- **Reflective practice** is required at all stages of the self-regulation cycle. Using as many different tools as appropriate information is gathered from a variety of sources, including personal and peer experiences, followed by a period of reflection that allows the individual to sort through the jumble of information and see how it fits in with their present understanding of their professional work. Where necessary present knowledge has to be deconstructed and then reconstructed into a new 'story' or understanding that takes into account any new information that the individual thinks is relevant. This new 'story' has to then be tried out, either by experimenting with it within the professional workplace or sharing it with peers. In either case the hoped-for outcome is 'improved practice', be it in terms of a skill or actual understanding. The outcome is then checked at the next self-audit stage of the self-regulation cycle.

If you just want to read one book...

Jenny Moon's book is an excellent outline for anyone wanting to find out more about this style of learning, with a good blend of theoretical background and practical ideas for developing the necessary skills:

Moon, J. (2004). *A Handbook of Reflective and Experiential Learning*. Oxon: RoutledgeFalmer.

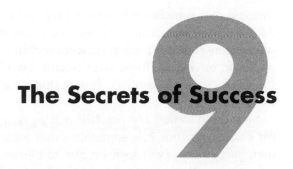

The Secrets of Success

Learning is our ticket to survival. (Weinstein, 1999)*

Most of us shared a raft of common values when we entered veterinary school: we decided that we wanted to become veterinarians because we cared about animals and we were looking for a respected and rewarding profession in the broadest sense of the word. We never expected to get rich fast, or to work weekdays only from nine to five, but we always felt that the veterinary profession could offer us so much more than those of our classmates who saw their future in careers such as banking, accountancy or the legal profession.

We were correct. Working as a practicing veterinarian does give us a totally unique opportunity to relate to animals and their

* Weinstein, K. (1999). *Action Learning – A Practical Guide*, 2nd edn. Aldershot: Gower. Reprinted with permission.

owners, and sometimes to make a real difference to their lives. Although hostile media comment occasionally comes our way, we are generally held in high esteem within our community, and are often envied by those who would have like to have had a career working with animals, but for one reason or another, never made it.

Success in veterinary practice will have a different meaning for each of us, but it is something that we all aspire to in our own particular way. It seems a pity to live our lives hoping that everything falls into place by chance, because as far as we know, we only have one shot at getting it right. Veterinary practice has all the key ingredients to allow us to fulfil all three of Martin Seligman's forms of happiness:

- A pleasant life
- An engaged life
- A meaningful life

Despite this the statistics demonstrate that a significant proportion of those that succeed in their goal of graduating as veterinarians become disillusioned with their work, leading to professional burn-out, psychological ill health, and in the most extreme cases, suicide.

The challenges of everyday veterinary practice are demanding on our time, and constantly being under pressure to provide information and make decisions is mentally exhausting. When we first qualify, it's generally all we can do to keep our heads above water and cope with what is thrown at us. As we progress through our careers, there is an understandable tendency to take the line of least resistance and remain in a reactive frame of mind, managing the challenges that face us, but largely at the mercy of external demands that seem outside of our control. A feeling of lack of control over our working environment contributes strongly to the sense of despair that results in long-term stress and sometimes breakdown.

In this book, I have firstly aimed to provide a framework to encourage veterinarians at any stage of their career to pause from the pressures of their work and think about some basic concepts. The earlier this is done, the better, and it is a process that is best repeated at regular intervals throughout our working lives. It involves:

- An examination of the beliefs and values that underlie our work ethic.
- A careful consideration of our life goals.
- A formulation of a clear personal vision that enables us and others around us to work towards the collection of goals that form our personal mission.
- Maintenance of a healthy balance between our work and the rest of our lives.

We are all well aware that there are clinical skills that we need to learn in order to practice effectively. As a profession, we are much less aware of the ancillary skills which have an equally powerful effect upon our ability to provide optimum patient care. Even when we are aware of them, we are much less likely to make an effort to develop them. These skills have been discussed in depth throughout this book but I now bring them together under five key areas that I consider to be crucial to developing good veterinary practice.

ATTITUDE

We are a caring profession, and it is axiomatic that good veterinary practice requires that we care. Caring about our patients is rarely an issue, since it is one of the core values that brings most of us into the profession. We also need to care about our clients, so must never forget that we work in a service industry, where a concern for clinical governance and quality of service is also of prime importance.

As a profession we fall down most frequently when it comes to caring for ourselves. We can only provide a lifetime of good veterinary practice within the context of a well-balanced and happy career, and if we fail to pay sufficient attention to that, our patients and our work colleagues will suffer in the long run. We need to constantly remind ourselves to approach our work with optimism and positivity, and appreciate that positive emotions bring positive results. We also need to balance our working lies with our social lives, and ensure we utilize our leisure time in a way that has the maximum positive effect upon our SWB.

Most of all, we need a passion for what we do, and for doing it well.

EMPATHY

Some of us are naturally empathetic and others have to work at it. The work of Daniel Goleman and others in this field has helped us to understand the nature and importance of emotional intelligence to our work. Small animal practice fuels the vast majority of the veterinary economy in all the Western countries, and that shows no sign of abating. Therefore, we need to recognize that a great deal of the profession's income hinges around one thing – the human/companion animal bond, so it is vital that we understand it and how it affects the behaviour of our clients. Obtaining the cooperation of our clients to carry out the treatments that are in the best interest of the animals in their charge is an essential part of successful veterinary practice, and it is most likely if a concordance between the recommendations of the veterinarian and the desires of the client is reached.

COMMUNICATIONS

Effective communications are vital at every interface that we have with those around us, including our work colleagues and our clients. We all tend to think that we communicate effectively, but a great proportion of the disciplinary and legal problems that arise from practice could have been avoided by better communications. The important starting point is that we need to recognize that communication skills are an important set of competencies, and that just like any others, they can be developed by a learning process.

LEADERSHIP

Most of us are instinctively drawn towards stability, but changes are inevitable, and it is vital that practices are able to react to them, anticipate them, or better still, initiate them. Effective leadership is about creating a work environment where good veterinary practice can thrive. Effective leaders do this by challenging the status quo, creating new visions and inspiring the workforce to fulfil their potential. In a service organization where the effective flow of knowledge is vital to success, it is essential that leadership skills are disseminated through the organization. Highly effective organizations generally have a much flatter hierarchical structure, with teams at the 'cutting edge' of service provision taking a greater level of responsibility for their actions.

The business models operating in the veterinary sphere are becoming more varied, with increased corporate ownership and joint venture partnerships, but the traditional partnership model still predominates in most areas. Veterinarians are not selected for entry to the profession primarily on the basis of their leadership and management skills, and so it is not surprising that practice principals do not always have either the skills or the inclination to be natural leaders or managers. In many instances it is the underlying strength of the market demand for veterinary services that has allowed poorly run practices to survive. The ultimate leadership of a veterinary practice does not have to lie in the hands of just one charismatic individual, and in reality it often does not, but it is vital that the practice owners recognize the need for effective leadership and formulate a strategy for ensuring that if the workforce have:

- Bought into a shared mission of where the practice is heading.
- Understood the practice goals that are required to work towards that mission, how they fit in with their personal goals and their role in fulfilling them.
- An awareness of, and broadly share, the values that underpin the way in which it functions.

Every veterinarian working in practice needs to be a leader to some degree. There are several different styles of leadership, and a really good leader will be able to call on more than one style to meet the demands of differing challenges. The most important characteristic is an ability to inspire the practice team, which requires a passion for what they do, good communication skills, a clear sense of vision and an empathetic understanding of what people desire and how to motivate them effectively.

The ultimate aim is to create a learning organization, where every member of the team is working together to constantly try and improve their performance. This requires the development of a no-blame culture.

> . . .*where people continually expand their capacity to create the results they truly desire, where new and expansive patterns of thinking are nurtured, where collective aspiration is set free, and where people are continually learning to see the whole together.* (Senge, 1990)

This objective is easy to state, but difficult to achieve, and extremely precious when it is fulfilled.

LEARNING AND REFLECTION

If continual learning is the key to successful veterinary practice, then reflection is the key to work-based learning. The product that we offer to our consumers is the output of the people who work within the organization. They are by far its most precious asset, and success in veterinary practice revolves around developing the competency of ourselves and those around us. In that way we can best meet the changing external forces that challenge us, and turn threats into opportunities.

The undergraduate veterinary course is extremely information-intensive, and although veterinary students are taught a great deal, there is insufficient emphasis upon developing one of life's most important skills – learning how to learn. This requires a self-awareness, an awareness of our own working environment, but also an advanced understanding of the nature of knowledge itself. Very little of our work is based upon incontrovertible truths, either due to gaps in the underlying knowledge base, or uncertainties that relate to the manner in which the knowledge is applied. Even when we are secure in advice that we offer, translating that into the predicted outcome brings with it yet another range of potential sources of error. We need to be able to strike a healthy balance between a healthy scepticism of the allegedly factual information that is fed to us, and the need for reasoned action.

As mature professionals, we need to develop the confidence to identify our own learning needs and then seek out the solutions to them, and to understand the styles of learning that best achieve the required objectives. We need to discriminate between the accumulation of knowledge, which is often best acquired as required ('just in time') rather than 'just in case', and true professional learning, which results in an improvement in the way in which we carry out our work. Time spent on reflection is very rarely time wasted, and we need to ensure that we allocate time from practice to develop our reflective processes. The technique of action learning in small peer groups that face a shared problem to solve can provide an excellent vehicle for this process.

It is easy for us to become defensive about what we do; our clients ostensibly pay us for giving them the 'correct' solutions to their problems, and the threat of legal or professional misconduct processes hangs over our heads. Yet those that think they carry out everything they do optimally are likely to be seriously deluded, and unable to critically examine what they do and how to do it more effectively. By developing those skills we can all not only continue to truly develop our careers, but even help to generate new knowledge from practice.

We live in a time of rapid change, which calls for entirely new ways of learning and thinking. In *Five Minds for the Future*, Howard Gardner defines the cognitive abilities that will command a premium in the years ahead:

- The disciplinary mind: Mastery of major schools of thought (including science, mathematics and history) and of at least one professional craft.
- The synthesizing mind: The ability to integrate ideas from different disciplines or spheres into a coherent whole and to communicate that integration to others.
- The creating mind: The capacity to uncover and clarify new problems, questions and phenomena.
- The respectful mind: Awareness of and appreciation for differences among human beings and human groups.

- The ethical mind: Fulfilment of one's responsibilities as a worker and citizen.

We are fortunate that the veterinary profession affords us the ability to develop all those aspects of our mental abilities, and so enjoy a meaningful life. But it is inevitable that at certain moments in our professional lives we will go through periods when we become disillusioned. The values that we upheld as important will have been subsumed by the realities of everyday veterinary life: not every case will involve overcoming a complex diagnostic challenge that saves the life of the animal involved and results in the undying gratitude of its owner. In fact, such cases are far and few between. Just as many may involve the frustration of not being able to take a diagnosis far enough due to practical constraints, or an owner that simply does not appreciate what is being done for them. Between these two extremes, the vast majority will be entirely commonplace, and superficially at least, unchallenging.

It is the routine that will make up the bulk of our working lives. Much of the clinical and management advice currently available has been written to help us cope with the extraordinary. That is perfectly valid: we need to know how to tackle the difficult clinical case: just as we need to know how to handle an unhappy and aggressive client. But as challenging as such instances may be, they are not the main factors that contribute to long-term professional dissatisfaction and burn-out: it's coping with the largely routine treadmill of professional life day after day, year after year, so we also need to know how to delight in the ordinary.

Success in veterinary practice does not require the attainment of perfection, but it is founded upon a passion for our work, and a commitment towards continual personal and professional development. Each of us will only be able to continue to perform to that standard if we develop our veterinary careers as part of a well-balanced life based upon sound values. Successful veterinary practice needs to be happy veterinary practice to thrive in the long term.

References

American Animal Hospital Association. (2003). *The Path to High Quality Healthcare – Practical Tips for Improving Compliance*. Colorado: AAHA Press.

Bartram, D.J. and Baldwin, D.S. (2007a). Veterinary surgeons and suicide: Influences, opportunities and research directions *Veterinary Record* 162, 36–40.

Bartram, D.J. and Boniwell, I. (2007b). The science of happiness: Achieving sustained psychological wellbeing. *In Practice* 29, 478–482.

Bartram, D.J. and Gardner, D. (2008). Coping with stress. *In Practice* 30, 228–231.

Bartram, D.J., Yadegarfar, G. and Baldwin, D.S. (2009). A cross-sectional study of mental heath and well-being and their associations in the UK veterinary profession. *Social Psychiatry and Psychiatric Epidemiology*. Available online; DOI 10.1007/s00127-009-0030-8.

Beanchamp, T. and Childress, J. (2001). *Principles of Biomedical Ethics*. Oxford: Oxford University Press.

Beckman, H.B. and Frankel, R.M. (1984). The effect of physician behavior upon the collection of data. *Annals of Internal Medicine* 101, 692–696.

Berwick, D.M. (1989). Continuous improvement as an ideal in health care. *New England Journal of Medicine* 320, 53–56.

Birks, Y. (2007). Emotional intelligence and patient-centred care. *JRSM* 100, 368–373.

Boniwell, I. (2006). *Positive Psychology in a Nutshell*. London: PWBC.

Brown, J. and Silverman, J. (1999). The current and future market for veterinarians and veterinary medical services in the United States. *JAVMA* 215, 161–183.

Brown, P. (2007). *Clinical Guidelines and the Veterinary Profession*. Masters thesis, Middlesex University.

Carnall, C. (1999). *Managing Change in Organizations*, 3rd edn. Harlow: Prentice Hall.

Carver, C.S. and Schier, M.F. (2002). Optimism. In *Handbook of Positive Psychology*. New York: Oxford University Press.

Charalambous, A. (2003). Reflective practice as a facilitator for learning. *Icus Nurse Web Journal*, Issue 13 January–March 2003. http://www.nursing.gr/reflectiveprac.pdf.

Cockcroft, P. and Holmes, M. (2003). *Evidenced Based Veterinary Medicine*. Oxford: Blackwell Publishing.

Csikszentmihalyi, M. (1992). *Flow: The Psychology of Happiness*. London: Rider.

David, A.J. (1990). *Total Quality Management and Business Excellence*, Vol. 1, Issue 1. London: Routledge.

Dembkowski, S., Eldridge, F. and Hunter, I. (2006). *The Seven Steps of Effective Executive Coaching*. London: Thorogood Publishing.

Diener, E. (1984). Subjective well-being. *Psychological Bulletin* 95 (3), 542–575.

Dreyfus, H.L. and Dreyfus, S.E. (1986). *Mind Over Machine: The Power of Human Intuition and Expertise in the Era of the Computer*. Oxford: Basil Blackwell.

Dunn, K. (2007). Editorial "looking back – moving forwards". *JSAP* 48 (1), 3.

Elkins, A.D. and Elkins, J.R. (1987). Professional burnout among US veterinarians: How serious a problem? *Veterinary Medicine* 82, 1245–1250.

Emmons, R.A. and McCullough, M.E. (2003). Counting blessings versus burdens: An experimental investigation of gratitude and subjective well-being in daily life. *Journal of Personality and Social Psychology* 84, 377–389.

Eraut, M. (1994). *Developing Professional Knowledge and Competence*. London: RoutledgeFalmer.

Evans, E., Louhiala, P. and Puustinen, R. (2004). *Philosophy for Medicine*. Oxford: Radcliffe Publishing.

Fleck, L. (1979). *Genesis and Development of a Scientific Fact*. Chicago: University of Chicago Press.

Ford, M.E. and Nichols, C.W. (1991). Using goals assessment to identify motivational patterns and facilitate behavioural regulation and achievement. *Advances in Motivation and Achievement* 7, 51–84.

Frankel, R.M. (2006). Pets, vets and frets: What relationship-centred care research has to offer veterinary medicine. *JVME* 33 (1), 20–27.

Fredrickson, B.L. (2001). The role of positive emotions in positive psychology: The broaden-and-build theory of positive emotions. *American Psychologist* 56, 218–226.

Fromm, E. (1976). *To Have or to Be?* New York: Continuum.

Gardner, H., Csikszentmihalyi, M. and Damon, W. (2006). *The Good Work Project – an Overview.* www.goodworkproject.org.

Garfield, C. (1986). *Peak Peformers: The New Heroes in Business.* London: Hutchinson Business.

Garvin, D.A. (1984). What does product quality really mean? *Sloan Management Review* 26, 45–43.

Goleman, D. (1995). *Emotional Intelligence: Why It Can Matter More Than IQ.* London: Sphere.

Goleman, D. (2000). *Leadership that gets results.* Harvard Business Review. Reprint R00204.

Goleman, D. (2007). *The New Leaders: Transforming the Art of Leadership into the Science of Results.* London: Sphere.

Hammond, K.R., McClelland, G.H. and Mumpower, J. (1980). *Human Judgment and Decision Making.* New York: Hemisphere.

Harr, R. (2001). TQM in dental practice. *International Journal of Health Care Quality Assurance* 14, 69–81.

Honey, P. and Mumford, A. (1982). *Manual of Learning Styles.* London: P. Honey.

Honey, P. and Mumford, A. (1993). *Using Your Learning Styles.* Maidenhead: Peter Honey Publications.

Horne, D. and Steadman-Jones, M. (2001). *Leadership: The Challenge for All?* London: Institute of Management/DTI/DEMOS.

Ioannidis, J.P.A. (2005). Why most published research findings are false. *PLoS Medicine* 2, e124.

Isaacs, D. and Fitzgerald, D. (1999). Seven alternatives to evidence based medicine. *BMJ* 319, 1618.

Isen, A., Rotzentzweig, A.S. and Young, M.J. (1991). The influence of positive effect on clinical problem solving. *Medical Decision Making* 11, 221–227.

Jevring-Bäck, C. (2007). *Managing a Veterinary Practice.* Edinburgh: Saunders Elsevier.

Keltner, D. and Bonanno, G.A. (1997). A study of laughter and dissociation: The distinct correlates of laughter and smiling during bereavement. *Journal of Personality and Social Psychology* 73, 687–702.

Kolb, D.A. (1984). *Experiential Learning: Experience As the Source of Learning and Development*. New Jersey: Prentice-Hall.

Leibovici, L. (2001). Effects of remote retroactive intercessory prayer on outcomes of patients with bloodstream infection: Randomized control trial. *BMJ* 323, 1450–1451.

Leighton, A. (2007). *On Leadership – Practical Wisdom form the People That Know*. London: Random House.

Lyuborminsky, S. (2001). Why are some people happier than others? The role of cognitive and motivational processes in well-being. *American Psychologist* 56 (3), 239–249.

Macan, T.H. (1996). Time management training: Effects on time behaviours, attitudes and job performance. *Journal of Psychology* 130, 229–237.

Manning, P. (2006). *Consultation Skills in Veterinary Practice*. Doctoral thesis, Middlesex University.

Maslow, A. (1999). *Toward a Psychology of Being*, 3rd edn. New York: Wiley.

McClelland, D. (1998). Indentifying competencies with behavioral-event interviews. *Psychological Science* 9, 331–339.

McGill, I. and Warner Weil, S. (1989). Continuing the new dialogue: New possibilities for experiential learning. In *Making Sense of Experiential Learning*. Milton Keynes, UK: Oxford University Press, pp. 24–74.

Mellanby, R.J. and Herrtage, M.E. (2004). Survey of mistakes made by recent veterinary graduates *Veterinary Record* 155, 761–765.

Mellanby, R.J., Crisp, J., De Palma, G., Spratt, D.P., Urwin, D., Wrght, M.J.H. et al. (2007). Perceptions of veterinarians and clients to expressions of clinical uncertainty. Editorial "looking back – moving forwards". *JSAP* 48 (1), 26–31.

Moon, J. (2004). *A Handbook of Reflective and Experiential Learning Oxon*. London: RoutledgeFalmer.

Moullin, M. (2002). *Delivering Excellence in Health and Social Care*. Buckingham: Open University Press.

National Institute for Clinical Excellence. (2002). *Principles for "Best Practice" in Clinical Audit*. Oxford, UK: Radcliffe Medical Press Ltd.

Neighbour, R. (2005). *The Inner Apprentice*, 2nd edn. Oxford: Radcliffe Publishing.

Nkanginieme, K.E.O. (1997). Clinical diagnosis as a dynamic cognitive process: Application of Bloom's taxonomy for educational objectives in the cognitive domain. *Medical Education* 2, 1. http://www.msu .edu/~dsolomon/f0000007.pdf.

Oishi, S., Diener, E., Suh, E. and Lucas, R.E. (1999). Value as a moderator in subjective well-being. *Journal of Personality* 67 (1), 157–184.

Pendleton, D. and Hasler, J. (eds). (1997). *Professional Development in General Practice.* Oxford: Oxford General Practice Series 37.

Persaud, R. (2005). *The Motivated Mind.* London: Bantam.

Pfeiffer, J.W., Goodstein, L.D. and Nolan, T.M. (1989). *Shaping Strategic Planning.* New York: University Associates Inc.

Poole, A.D. and Sanson-Fisher, R.W. (1979). Understanding the patient: A neglected aspect of medical education. *Social Science and Medicine* 13A, 37.

Rodin, J. (1986). Aging and health: Effects of the sense of control. *Science* 233, 1271–1276.

Rogers, C.R. (1961). *On Becoming a Person: The Struggle Towards Self-Realization.* London: Constable, p. 351

Rowe, M.B. (1986). Wait time: Slowing down may be a way of speeding up. *Journal of Teacher Education* 37, 43–50.

Royal College of Nursing. (1996). *Clinical Effectiveness Strategy.* London: Royal College of Nursing.

Ryan, R.M. and Deci, E.L. (2000). Self determination theory and the facilitation of intrinsic motivation, and well-being. *American Psychologist* 55, 68–78.

Ryan, R.M. and Deci, E.L. (2001). On happiness and human potentials: A review o f research on hedonic and eudaemonic well-being. *Annual Review of Psychology* 52, 141–166.

Sackett, D.L, Richardson, W.S. Rosenberg, W. and Haynes, B.R. (1997). *Evidence-Based Medicine: How to Practice and Teach EBM.* Edinburgh: Churchill Livingstone.

Saunders, J. (2004). Do we really have to live with this? Uncertainty in medicine. In *Philosophy for Medicine*, M. Evans, P. Louhiala and R. Puustinen (eds). Oxford: Radcliffe Medical Press.

Scally, G. and Donaldson, L.J. (1998). Clinical governance and the drive for quality improvement in the New NHS in England. *BMJ* 317 (7150), 61–65.

Schön, D.A. (1983). *The Reflective Practitioner: How Professionals Think in Action.* London: Temple Smith.

Seligman, M.E.P. (1991). *Learned Optimism.* New York: Knopf.

Seligman, M.E.P. (2002). *Authentic Happiness.* New York: The Free Press.

Seligman, M.E.P. (2005). Positive psychology progress: Empirical validation of interventions. *American Psychologist* 60, 410–421.

Senge, P. (1990). *The Fifth Discipline: The Art and Practice of the Learning Organization*. London: Random House.

Senge, P., Berchtold, S. and Zehetmayr, U. (1999). *The Dance of Change*. London: Nicholas Brealey Publishing.

Shuttleworth, S. (2006). *Developing a Strategy to Validate Veterinary Professional Practice*. Doctoral thesis, National Centre for Work Based Learning Partnerships, Middlesex University.

Shuttleworth, S.C. (2003). *What Skills Will Veterinary General Practitioners Need to Develop in Order to Meet Future Opportunities and Threats to the Profession?* MSc thesis. www.vetgp.co.uk.

Shwartz, S.H. (1994). Are there universal aspects in the content and structure of values? *Journal of Social Issues* 50, 19–46.

Silverman, J., Kurtz, S. and Draper, J. (1998). *Skills for Communicating with Patients*. Oxon: Radcliffe Medical Press.

Silverman, J., Kurtz, S. and Draper, J. (2004). *Teaching and Learning Communication Skills in Medicine*. Oxon: Radcliffe Medical Press.

Smith, R. (1992). Audit and research. *BMJ* 305, 905–906.

Smith, R. (1994). Medicine's core values. *BMJ* 309, 1247–1248.

Smith, R. (2006). *The Trouble with Medical Journals*. London: RSM Press.

Snyder, C.R., Rand, K.L. and Sigmon, D.R. (2002). Hope theory: A member of the positive psychology family. In *Handbook of Positive Psychology*. New York: Oxford University Press, pp. 257–266.

SPVS Masters Group. (2003). The 'masters group' survey: Progress on new GP qualification. *Veterinary Times* 12th May, 22–23.

Storey, J. (2004). *Leadership in Organizations: Current Issues and Key Trends*. London: Routledge.

Sumedho, A. (1995). *The Mind and the Way: Buddhist Reflections on Life*. Boston: Wisdom Publications.

Tuckett, D., Boulton, M., Olsen, C. and Williams, A. (1985). *Meetings Between Experts: An Approach to Sharing Ideas in Medical Consultations*. London: Tavistock.

Viner, B. (2003). *Attitudes to Clinical Auditing in Veterinary General Practice*. Masters thesis, Middlesex University.

Viner, B. (2006). *Introducing to Clinical Audit in Veterinary Practice*. Doctorate thesis, Middlesex University.

Viner, B. (2009). Using audit to improve clinical effectiveness. In *Practice*, Vol. 31, No. 5. London: BVA Publications.

Warr, P. (2007). *Work, Happiness and Unhappiness*. London: LEA Publishers.

Weinstein, K. (1999). *Action Learning – A Practical Guide*, 2nd edn. Aldershot: Gower.

Welch, J. (1996). Letter to shareholders. In *General Electric Annual Report,* Stamford.

Williams, S.M., Arnold, P.K. and Mills, J.N. (2005). Coping with stress: A survey of Murdoch University Veterinary students. *Journal of Veterinary Medical Education* 32, 201–212.

Index